THE PCOS DIE

OTHER TITLES IN THIS SERIES:
by the same author:
PCOS: A Woman's Guide to Dealing with Polycystic Ovary Syndrome
(Colette Harris with Dr Adam Carey)

THE PCOS DIET BOOK

HOW YOU CAN USE
THE NUTRITIONAL APPROACH
TO DEAL WITH
POLYCYSTIC OVARY SYNDROME

Colette Harris
and Theresa Cheung

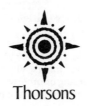

Thorsons

Thorsons
An Imprint of HarperCollins*Publishers*
77–85 Fulham Palace Road,
Hammersmith, London W6 8JB

The Thorsons website address is: www.thorsons.com

are trademarks of
HarperCollins*Publishers* Limited

Published by Thorsons 2002

3 5 7 9 10 8 6 4

A catalogue record for this book
is available from the British Library

ISBN 0 00 713184 4

Printed in Great Britain by
Martins the Printers Ltd, Berwick-upon-Tweed

Contents

Acknowledgements

Colette:

I want to say a heartfelt thank you to my partner Chris for his constant interest in my work, his patient and skilful reading of the manuscript, and his help keeping me practising what I preach so I stay on top of my own PCOS, and my family and friends for their support.

I am very grateful to Dr Ann Walker for her reading of the manuscript and enthusiastic Foreword, but also for her generous interest and belief in this book. A big thank you also to all the experts quoted who gave time and thought to the questions asked, and shared their knowledge; to Wanda Whiteley at Thorsons for all her help and patience, and to Megan Slyfield at Thorsons for her dedication and support, and to Barbara Vesey for her patience and skill.

Special thanks to all the women with PCOS who donated their stories and spent time talking to us about emotional subjects – your stories throughout the book are a source of comfort and inspiration.

Finally a huge and special tribute to Theresa for her fantastic energy, enthusiasm and unwavering professionalism – it has been a joy to work on this project with you.

Theresa:

Thank you to my husband Ray and to my two beautiful children Robert and Ruth for their patience, support and love while I completed this project. Thanks also to my brother Terry, his partner Robin, and the support of family and friends.

Thank you to the many experts and advisors, especially Helen Mason, Sally Wharmby, Claire Mellors, Judith Verity and Sophie Elkan, and all the women with PCOS who talked to me during the writing of this book. I am truly grateful for the insight they gave me.

Thank you to our editor, Wanda Whiteley, for her encouragement, support and advice and for putting me in touch with Colette to work on this project. Finally a big thank you to Colette for her commitment, dedication, insight and her amazing ability to make even the most complex medical and academic jargon easy to understand. Above all I would like to thank her for her kindness, understanding and respect. It has been a pleasure to work with her every step of the way.

Medical Disclaimer

The therapies and treatments described in this book are not intended to replace the services of a trained health professional. Your own physical condition and diagnosis may require specific modifications and precautions. Before undertaking any treatment or therapy you should consult your physician or health care provider. Special precautions may be required if you are on medication for PCOS or under treatment for diabetes, infertility, thyroid disorder or depression.

Any application of the ideas, suggestions and procedures set forth in this book are at the reader's discretion.

Foreword

We now know that PCOS is a common condition that must have plagued women for generations. Only a decade ago it was barely recognized by medical practitioners, and most women would have suffered their symptoms in silence. At last, with greater understanding of its underlying causes, PCOS is now being taken seriously. Much of the credit for greater public awareness in the UK goes to Colette Harris and her previous book *PCOS: A Woman's Guide to Dealing with Polycystic Ovary Syndrome* and for her tireless support for Verity, the PCOS support group.

As a scientist, nutritionist and medical herbalist I am impressed by how far Colette Harris and Theresa Francis-Cheung have delved into the scientific and medical literature to review what is currently known about PCOS and its treatment. In this book they present the information in an easy-to-read form, together with the voices of PCOS sufferers, with whom many women will identify. Sufferers can now see a rational basis for their diverse symptoms, founded on poor utilization of insulin. For example, this new concept goes a long way to explain why weight loss is so difficult for women with PCOS.

But help is at hand!

This book is full of tips on diet and lifestyle changes that can help the body to use insulin more efficiently. It shows how the vicious cycle of weight gain, with increasing difficulty of weight loss, can be broken, and that the debilitating and embarrassing signs and symptoms of PCOS really can disappear.

There is no doubt that, both from clinical data and from my own experience as a practitioner, switching to a healthy diet and adopting a healthy lifestyle would make a huge difference to the well-being of many people in the Western world. However, even with due attention to diet, many women do not reach their recommended target intakes for vitamins and minerals while on weight-reducing regimes. This is the dilemma faced by many women with PCOS, and is where nutrient supplements can be so very helpful. While they should never be a substitute for healthy eating, vitamin and mineral nutrition supplements can be used in conjunction with a good diet to ensure optimal nutrition of the key organs of the body involved in hormone balance.

Valuable guidance is given in this book on appropriate nutrient supplements, together with herbs that may be used to speed the way to health. However, since sufficient detail on the use of herbs cannot be conveyed in a book such as this, women with PCOS would benefit greatly from consulting a professional. If you want to consult a Medical Herbalist, look for the qualifications MNIMH or FNIMH (Member or Fellow of the National Institute of Medical Herbalists, UK) or MCPP (Member of the College of Practitioners of Phytotherapy, UK). These practitioners have had four years of rigorous medical training and will give sympathetic advice on PCOS. The addresses of these organizations are given at the back of the book.

There is no need to suffer in silence these days – if you have PCOS you can choose to have health and well-being. Although it will involve some effort, by following the advice given in this book you can make a positive difference to your own health and take control of your life again. It is an excellent guide to our current state of knowledge and is written from an integrated medical perspective by an ex-sufferer.

Dr Ann Walker PhD MNIMH MCPP
Senior Lecturer in Human Nutrition
Hugh Sinclair Unit of Human Nutrition School of Food Biosciences
The University of Reading, UK
27 September 2001

Introduction

I admit it – I'm nosy. When I'm in the supermarket I can't help peering into other people's trolleys. And you can tell a lot about a person from what they buy – the single man with his beer and ready-meals, the girlfriends settling in for a good night of chatting with their Chardonnay and chocolates, the woman with a trolley full of food for her family, with fizzy drinks, crisps and pizzas alongside the fruit and veg and milk and cereal, the woman shopping for herself and her partner, stuffing in his favourite cuts of meat, cheese and bread for sandwiches that she'll end up eating too. What isn't so easy to spot is what impact that food will have on our health when we eat it day after day.

For the one in ten women who has PCOS – and consider that half of them don't even know it yet – many of the daily food choices of the average Western diet stacked high in supermarkets will damage their health now and make them more likely to get diabetes in the future. I'm one of those women. And I realized how vital taking control of my diet was when I developed debilitating symptoms of PCOS after coming off the Pill aged 23. Slowly but surely my hair started falling out faster and faster, an overwhelming fatigue took over my body, leaving me needing to sleep for 18 hours a day at weekends, unwanted hairs sprouted on my upper lip and abdomen, and livid, tender, lumpy spots became routine, instead of occasional PMS visitors, all over my face, back and upper chest. My periods got less frequent until they dwindled to nothing – my weight, on the other hand, crept steadily upwards. And let's not even get started on those mood swings!

After a long drawn-out process of repeated visits to the doctor I managed to get blood tests and an ultrasound scan that gave me the PCOS diagnosis, but when I asked about treatments other than the Pill (I'd never felt well on the several brands I had tried, with regular fainting bouts, dizziness, hot flushes and bloating) I was referred to a gynaecologist with a five-month wait and told they wouldn't know anything else really, either, but I could go if I really wanted to.

I was faced with the prospect of five more months of declining health, or taking matters into my own hands. I decided to turn PCOS-detective.

At that time there weren't any really user-friendly websites, no support groups, no books other than medical texts and medical studies which were full of difficult jargon. I was – and still am – in the privileged position to be working for the UK's leading natural health magazine, *Here's Health*, with access to a fantastic library and a network of complementary health experts who seemed to know a fair amount about treating women with PCOS. Using their expertise, trawling through books and every website I could find with any useful information on it, I decided to become my own guinea pig and started eating a very healthy vegetarian diet, with very, very little alcohol, caffeine or high-fat dairy foods, plenty of soy, wholegrains, fruits and vegetables and taking the herb agnus castus as well as other supplements including essential fatty acids. I also had reflexology treatment and did a naturopathic detox.

I was amazed to find that within six weeks my periods were back, my hair was thicker and my spots were vanishing. I was convinced that food was the missing link in treating PCOS. Five years later, this book proves that it really is – the volume of research and scientific interest in PCOS and diet has grown massively over the last few years – there are now support groups and websites, discussion groups and chat rooms, and a whole lot more openness about PCOS and its sometimes embarrassing symptoms. But what hasn't been shouted from the rooftops enough is the fact that eating a balanced, healthy diet with a few PCOS-tailored twists will not only help you beat your symptoms but it will protect your future health. Because PCOS isn't just about the day-to-day grind of spots, tiredness, weight gain and wondering when your next period will arrive. The hard facts are that it's about being at an increased risk of diabetes, heart disease, high blood pressure and fertility problems in the long term. And although a lot of medication can help you deal with your symptoms day to day – the simplest, most effective way to cut your risks for all these conditions and boost your fertility into the bargain is to eat well and exercise.

This has to be one of the most satisfying things for me about managing my PCOS using diet as the essential basis for good health. It's something simple I can do every day to help myself feel better – and after the long haul of trying to get a diagnosis for my symptoms, and trying to come to terms with having this lifelong condition, it was one of the most fantastic feelings to be able to take control again with the simple act of cooking myself nourishing meals.

It almost sounds too simple – and maybe some of you are thinking 'Oh no, not another healthy eating plan, I've heard it all before.' But what's different about this book is that it's tailored for PCOS and explains exactly why each step of the healthy eating programme we suggest is good for helping to deal with this condition.

What's more, it's not just a healthy eating plan. Just as there's far more to PCOS than weight problems, there's also far more to healthy eating than knowing why you should eat specific foods. Being a health journalist and a woman who uses diet and natural medicine to manage her own PCOS, I can truly understand that massive gap between knowing what's good for you and actually getting round to doing it! Every day I read and write about why healthy living can boost energy, radiance and vitality – and yet sometimes all I want to do is crawl home and eat my way through a bath of melted chocolate.

This emotional relationship with food is at the core of any healthy eating plan. I'm really pleased at having got so far into eating well that it's now a habit, not a chore, and I truly enjoy fresh, flavoursome food. But on those odd miserable, stressed or PMS nights there's practically nothing that can stop me munching on chocolate or plum bread or malt loaf or soggy toast with raspberry jam – what I want is to feel treated and cozy and glad to be home where I can hibernate and forget the day. And I think the key to my ability to keep committed to healthy eating is as much to do with getting rid of guilt when I do pig out as with the knowledge that eating well will help me beat PCOS. If you're eating well most of the time, the odd treat isn't going to kill you, and it's taken me a long time to get to feel so balanced about my food.

Like many women with PCOS, I went through a difficult time with food. At 19 and under 9 stone and 5 ft 10 inches tall, my doctor recommended I should get up to an ideal weight of 10 stone and a few pounds. The idea horrified me. I couldn't bear to think of allowing my tight control over my body weight and food intake to diminish, because I instinctively felt that if I let it slip even a tiny bit I'd start eating all the chocolate, puddings and sweet foods I loved, and balloon into someone I just didn't want to be.

When I discovered I had PCOS years later and began to understand why having a slower metabolism and insulin resistance can cause the easy weight gain that accompanies the condition, the pieces began to fall into place. Once I got my herbal medicine and nutritional supplements programme going, and started to really make an effort to eat more healthy organic food every day, deal with stress better and detox my lifestyle, my PCOS symptoms – and a lot of the extra weight I had put on – slowly melted away.

Ideas about what a healthy diet is and why you should eat it are all too often linked to starvation, denial and ludicrous ideas about what an 'ideal body weight' would be. As a woman in a world which all too often equates attractiveness and success with the size and shape of your body, I'm all too aware of those fad diets promising instant glamour, and as a woman with PCOS who struggles with her weight I'm also aware of how tempting it can be to try them.

But PCOS is about a lot more than controlling your weight. Losing weight – if you really do have weight to lose – can help, and your diet does have a part to play in that. But how many of us have complained about unsympathetic doctors telling us that our weight is the problem and if we lose it our symptoms and fertility will sort themselves out? Your PCOS diet can be about so much more than weight loss! I have been amazed to discover the healing power of the foods I've eaten over the five years since I was diagnosed, and to learn that food doesn't have to be the enemy. Its active healing compounds can actually be a huge part of beating your symptoms, staying well and protecting your health well into the future.

Just to put the record straight, I can assure you that healthy, fresh foods are not always more expensive than 'convenience' foods – in fact, they're often cheaper if you buy from markets and greengrocers. What they may cost you is a bit of extra time to prepare when you first start out.

What this book will show you is that eating a truly healthy diet for PCOS is about nourishing your body with all the vital vitamins, minerals and other nutrients it needs in order to create hormonal balance and normalize insulin reactions. This helps to beat symptoms now, boost fertility, protect you from diabetes and heart disease in the future and even helps whatever medical or natural health care you use for your PCOS to work more effectively.

In other words, eating a healthy diet – in conjunction with a basic exercise plan – is a win-win situation for women with PCOS. And the best thing about this is that *you're* the person who can make it happen every day.

I truly hope that this book, which Theresa and I have written knowing what it is to have PCOS, will help you to start seeing food as an essential ally in the fight to manage this condition.

If we can do it, so can you!

Colette Harris
May 2002

Part One

NUTRITIONAL HEALING FOR PCOS –

LAYING THE FOUNDATIONS

Why Food Is So Important for Women with PCOS

There's no denying that food is important. It gives you the energy you need to get through the day, tantalizes you with enjoyable tastes and feeds your body with the essential goodness it needs to work properly.

Study after study proves that good nutrition is the foundation of good health, and the ideal way to stay healthy and fit – whether you have PCOS or not. Everyone should try to eat more fruit and vegetables, reduce their fat intake, eat less high-sugar and high-salt foods and steer clear of the dessert trolley in restaurants. But once you are diagnosed with PCOS and you enter the 'no woman's land' where no one is quite sure what the condition is, what causes it and what is the right way to cure it (see Appendix), the one thing that has been proven time and time again is that *a healthy diet is of enormous value.*

Food can play an important medical role in helping to deal with PCOS. Many of the symptoms – from weight problems, skin condition and energy levels to menstrual patterns, acne and excess facial and body hair – can all be improved by eating the right foods and, more importantly, by avoiding those which aren't going to be helpful. With this book you'll learn how to design a diet that can help you restore blood-sugar levels, balance your hormones, improve energy levels, lose weight and address any PCOS symptoms you may have.

So why is food such a powerful tool when you have PCOS? Why is a healthy diet actually the first essential step – in combination with exercise – to managing the condition, keeping the symptoms at bay and enhancing the effects of any medication you decide to take?

> **Polycystic Ovary Syndrome (PCOS) is a condition caused by hormonal imbalance and insulin resistance which leads to symptoms such as weight gain, excess body hair, acne and irregular or absent periods. (For a fuller description of PCOS as a medical condition, read Appendix.)**

THE INSULIN LINK

The first reason food is so important for PCOS is its direct impact on our hormonal system. All the food we eat evokes a hormonal response in our bodies. Since PCOS is a health condition linked with hormonal imbalances and – as the latest research suggests – insulin resistance[1] (a precursor state to diabetes), food may well be the cheapest and most effective medicine available.

Many women with PCOS have high levels of insulin in their blood, a condition called *hyperinsulinism*. Insulin is a peptide hormone (a small protein made from a string of amino acids) made by the pancreas. It controls blood-sugar levels by allowing the body's cells to take up and use glucose (sugar) for energy.

Normally when a meal is eaten, the pancreas releases insulin into the bloodstream to encourage the body's cells to store away or use the energy released from the meal.

If the body's cells don't respond to the insulin, they are described as 'insulin resistant' – 'hard of hearing' to insulin's message. To make the cells hear the message, the body has to turn up the volume by increasing the amount of insulin the pancreas makes for a given amount of glucose in the blood.

The problem with high levels of insulin is that they stimulate the ovaries to produce large amounts of male hormones known as androgens, of which testosterone is the most powerful and well known. Excess androgens are thought to stop the ovaries releasing an egg, causing irregular or absent periods – one of the most common symptoms of PCOS. High testosterone levels in women also cause acne, male-pattern baldness and excess hair growth. Last, but not least, it is the insulin problem, combined with high levels of androgen, which puts women with PCOS at increased risk of diabetes as well as heart disease.

You can eat in a way that helps to reduce insulin resistance and make your body's cells more responsive again. The health benefits of a diabetes diet to regulate blood-sugar levels are well known. When you have diabetes, your main concern is always how what you eat affects your blood-sugar and insulin levels. Since insulin resistance and excess androgen are strongly linked to PCOS, the key to treating or avoiding PCOS through nutrition is to achieve balanced blood-sugar levels while nourishing your body in such a way that it can maintain an appropriate balance of hormones.

Changing my diet changed my life. It took being diagnosed with PCOS for me to fully appreciate the incredible impact food can have on my health and my symptoms. I've really learned the hard way that you are what you eat.
Samantha, 36

Once I started to make the connection between the food I was eating and my symptoms, I saw a remarkable improvement in my symptoms. I lost weight and I lost the cravings I had when my blood sugar dropped. Best of all, I got my energy back.
Diana, 40

EATING TO HELP WEIGHT CONTROL

A second reason food can be a powerful tool for managing PCOS is its role in weight control. How much you weigh and the amount of body fat you have are two of the most important factors in determining how severe your symptoms of PCOS are. Repeated studies show that losing weight can result in improvements.[2] Many of us with PCOS know only too well that this can be really difficult (more on that in a moment), but weight loss – if you are presently overweight – can really help.

Research shows that overweight women with PCOS have more fertility problems than lean women with PCOS.[3] Overweight women with PCOS who diet and lose weight find that their testosterone levels fall and PCOS symptoms diminish. The weight loss doesn't have to be dramatic, either. Some women lost just a few pounds, others lost much more. In both cases weight loss lead to remarkable improvements in fertility: 82 per cent of the women who were not previously ovulating ovulated, with a number of successful pregnancies, even though these women had had long-standing histories of infertility.

No one really knows why PCOS responds so well to weight loss. It may be linked with the fact that overweight women (without PCOS) can dramatically increase their fertility by losing weight.[4] It may also be that weight loss lowers insulin levels, which in turn reduces the ovaries' production of testosterone. When you gain weight, levels of insulin and testosterone increase; the hormonal chaos this creates can make symptoms of PCOS worse. It could also be because fat itself gives out more oestrogen, adding to the hormonal imbalance.

Whatever the reason, avoiding anything that can trigger weight gain, insulin resistance and an overproduction of male hormones is important in helping to manage PCOS symptoms.

In addition to a reduction in severity of symptoms, there is another reason why weight loss is a really positive step for overweight women with PCOS. If you have PCOS you are more likely than those without to have weight-management problems. Research shows that obesity is four times more likely in women who have PCOS and irregular periods than those without.[5] The tendency in women with PCOS is to put on weight around the waist rather than the hips – making for an apple shape as opposed to a pear shape.[6] In a recent review, PCOS expert Professor Gabor T Kovacs from Monash Medical School, Box Hill Hospital, Melbourne, Australia cites studies that confirm that 'Women with PCOS appear to remain centrally obese when approaching the menopause.'[7]

Gaining weight around the middle is associated with a higher risk of poor health according to a 25-year study at Gothenburg University in Sweden. No one is really sure why being an 'apple' carries with it more health risks than being a pear, but it may be due to the way the body processes fat stored in different parts of the body. Fat around the tummy is constantly being broken down and circulated around the body, while fat around the bottom is not. Higher levels of circulating fat increase the risk of heart disease and narrowing of the arteries. Abdominal fat can also put pressure on internal organs such as the heart.

With insulin resistance and excess weight already putting a strain on the heart, the fat-distribution problem is another incentive for keeping to a healthy weight if you have PCOS.

So is losing weight the answer? Unfortunately it isn't that simple.

THE PCOS METABOLISM – WHY DIETS DON'T WORK

It's the weight gain that's caused me most problems. I used to joke about being fat but inside I felt miserable and desperate. At my biggest I rocketed up to 16 stone 3 lb. I'm trapped in a vicious cycle. I know that losing weight will improve my symptoms, but I'm finding it virtually impossible.
Catherine, 30

If you have always felt you only need look at food to put on weight, your feelings are shared by many women with PCOS. You may have tried to diet and found it doesn't work in the long run. At first you might see an improvement, but soon, the more you restrict your calories the more your body goes into starvation mode, conserving even more energy and storing away the calories it does get as fat reserves in case the 'starvation' carries on. You eventually reach a point where dieting doesn't seem to help you lose weight.

If you have PCOS, in addition to your body's typical reaction to restricted food intake you have another hurdle to face: women with PCOS store fat more efficiently and burn up calories more slowly than women who don't have PCOS, even when they're not on a diet.

I stopped having periods when I was about 17. My doctor put me on the Pill to balance my hormones. I have always been a little overweight. I used to be able to lose weight by dieting, but in the last few years however hard I try I just can't shift the weight. It isn't fair. I eat the same as my skinny friends but I'm putting on weight. And the fatter I get, the more facial hair I get. There are days when I just can't face the world and want to hide from everyone.
Emma, 33

Your *metabolic rate* is the rate at which your body burns calories. The faster your metabolic rate, the more you can eat without putting on weight. The slower your metabolic rate, the more you need to watch your food intake. Metabolic rate is increased by any form of activity, including eating. The rate at which food is metabolized after a meal is called *postprandial thermogenesis*.

For most people, postprandial thermogenesis accounts for a large percentage of their daily calorie burning. But studies show that postprandial thermogenesis in women with PCOS is significantly reduced.[8] Basically, after you eat a meal your body doesn't burn up the calories as quickly as it would if you didn't have PCOS. Your slower metabolism means you store more calories from the food you eat.

And if you have PCOS and insulin resistance, you also have to deal with the consequence of insulin preventing you from burning the calories off. According to Dr Richard S Legro in the *American Journal of Obstetrics and Gynecology*, women with PCOS showed as much as a 40 per cent lower response to the stress hormones that trigger the breakdown of fat than did healthy women, whether or not the PCOS women were obese.[9]

So not only does being overweight make you more likely to develop an increasing number and severity of symptoms, but if you have polycystic ovaries you are more likely to put on weight.

The PCOS Catch-22

The inability to lose weight can lead to stress, which in turn leads to comfort eating. You can end up feeling trapped in a vicious cycle, with the pounds piling on.

Losing weight can be frustrating if you have PCOS, but by making specific changes in your diet and the *way* you eat it is possible to regain control of the situation, to maintain or lose weight and feel good about yourself. Hopefully this book will help you make weight-management problems a thing of the past.

SELF-HELP SATISFACTION

Another reason food is so important if you have PCOS is that it is something you can control. A feeling of powerlessness can be overwhelming if you are dealing with a long-term health condition which requires visits to health-care practitioners and involves dealing daily with unpleasant and disheartening symptoms. The symptoms of PCOS (see Appendix) can often strike at the heart of your femininity and batter your self-esteem. Many women have experienced unhelpful attitudes from health-care practitioners who have simply insisted that losing weight is the key to better health with PCOS, without understanding the difficulties this involves.

My doctor told me that if I wanted to improve my symptoms I would need to lose weight. As if I hadn't been trying all those years! Did he think I wanted to look and feel like this? I can't remember a day of my life when I haven't been dieting, restricting calories or exercising to burn calories, but nobody believes me. They all think I don't have enough will-power or discipline to lose weight.
Lucy, 34

Feeling powerless, hopeless and not listened to can be crushing psychologically and make you feel low and depressed. Changing your diet can transform your feelings of powerlessness into a more positive outlook, because it's something you can take charge of every day.

I remember being showed the scan and seeing dark blobs around my ovaries. I was told that I had polycystic ovary syndrome and this was causing my irregular periods, acne and weight gain. 'That's it,' I thought, 'I'm going to be fat and spotty for the rest of my life.' I felt completely hopeless until my doctor told me that I could, to a certain extent, control my symptoms through my diet. I wasn't at the mercy of my hormones. There was something I could do to help myself.
Clare, 28

Since the age of 9 I started to gain weight uncontrollably. I became very depressed and lost a lot of confidence. I got my first period when I was 12, but after one or two more they stopped. I went to doctor after doctor and they all blamed my lack of periods on my weight. This made me feel even more depressed. It wasn't until last year that a fertility specialist diagnosed me with PCOS. I have all the classic symptoms – high insulin, weight gain, rough dry skin, acne, excess body and facial hair and just about every other thing that can make me feel like a boy rather than a girl.

When I was diagnosed I was relieved, but I was also angry. Why was this happening to me? I asked my doctor what I could do and he said that I should visit a dietician with specialist knowledge of PCOS to design a diet which could control my insulin levels. That was the incentive I needed. The weight started to come off and it gave me the confidence to start exercising and make other lifestyle choices, like stopping smoking, drinking less and taking multivitamins, which ease my symptoms.

Looking back, I think PCOS has made me a stronger person. It has helped me understand that the most important thing in life is your health. A lot of people don't realize how many risks they are taking with their health when they don't eat well. But I do.
Bryony, 17

Eating well is something you can do every day to nourish your body and mind. The positive lift you get from feeling that every day you are doing something to alleviate your PCOS symptoms, boost your energy and enhance the power of any medication you may be taking is a great feeling to have when you're battling with so many emotions. Having a daily dose of self-help on a plate is really energizing and motivating.

Eating healthily every day gives you the opportunity to re-invent yourself. With every breath you take, every meal you eat, every drink you swallow, you are literally building a new you by supplying your body with the raw materials it needs to repair your skin, generate new tissues, balance hormones and create more cells. Your food is the building block to better health.

So every day, as you feed your body with what it needs to work at its peak of health, remind yourself that you deserve the best. Many women with PCOS notice striking improvements when they take matters into their own hands and embark on the right diet and exercise plan.

Remember: If you have PCOS, what you eat or don't eat is absolutely crucial and, more importantly, within your control.

GETTING WHAT YOU NEED

Food isn't just important to women with PCOS because it helps with insulin resistance and gives you back a feeling of control over your health. Food is also vital because it contains essential nutrients which the human body needs in order to function properly.

Nutritional deficiencies – when you don't get enough of all the essential vitamins, minerals and other nutrients you need to keep your body running efficiently – can be caused by diet or outside forces like stress and pollution, which make your body use up more nutrients in order to protect itself. Nutritional deficiencies can disturb the whole intricate system of your body.

As well as having a role in the struggle against diseases such as cancer, arthritis and heart disease, diet can also help combat infertility, stress, insomnia and conditions like PMS.

The aim of nutritional therapy tailored for PCOS, and the role of a nutritional therapist – someone trained to see food and nutritional supplements as medicine, and help you to use them to correct imbalances in the body – would be to reduce insulin levels by lowering blood-sugar and other triggers of insulin production, such as stimulants like coffee and stress. Eating the right kinds of food can provide the body with the proper nutrients so it can correct the underlying hormonal imbalances which lie at the root of PCOS, and tackle specific symptoms such as sugar cravings, acne, hair loss, irregular periods and depression.

For instance, avoiding saturated fat and high-sugar foods, and increasing fibre intake, can help to reduce androgen levels and ease the symptoms which are triggered when male hormones are out of balance.

Many women with PCOS also have to deal with 'unopposed' oestrogen, which occurs when no ovulation takes place in a menstrual cycle, so that there is no surge of progesterone in the second half of the cycle to balance out the normal levels of oestrogen. Unopposed oestrogen can cause symptoms such as hot sweats and dizziness. Dietary changes such as avoiding junk foods and unhealthy carbohydrates and ensuring an adequate intake of essential fatty acids and healthy carbohydrates would aim to restore the correct balance of oestrogen, progesterone and androgen. (See Chapter 2 for descriptions of healthy and unhealthy carbohydrates.)

According to clinical nutritionist Conner Middleman Whitney, who has studied and documented the effects of nutritional therapy on PCOS via a three-month internet study involving dietary changes and nutritional supplements, 'More work needs to be done into the link between nutrition and PCOS. However, for women seeking to overcome the many symptoms associated with PCOS, I strongly believe that nutritional therapy can offer powerful support.'[10]

PROTECT YOUR FUTURE HEALTH

Making simple and beneficial changes to your diet and lifestyle are the first important steps towards balanced hormones and a state of good, natural health. But what about protecting your health in the years to come?

If you have PCOS, you are potentially at a higher risk of developing the following long-term health problems:

Obesity
Many women with PCOS find that their symptoms get worse when they put on weight. Being overweight has many long-term associated health problems. It reduces mobility, prolongs healing time and increases the risks of all the other long-term health conditions listed below.

Infertility
This is defined as an inability to conceive after one year of regular unprotected sex. PCOS causes problems with ovulation due to imbalances in the hormones LH (luteinizing hormone) and FSH (follicle stimulating hormone). If a woman isn't ovulating she can't conceive, so PCOS is linked to infertility. But some women with PCOS ovulate, some ovulate occasionally, and others are only ever infertile for the odd month or two.

Miscarriage
This is the loss of a pregnancy, normally before 14 weeks. Women with PCOS, who have high levels of Luteinizing Hormone, may be at greater risk of early pregnancy loss. Of women with recurrent miscarriage, more than 80 per cent have been identified as having polycystic ovaries.

Eating disorders
A recent study suggested that PCO/S does not cause eating disorders,[11] but since many women with PCOS

have problems controlling their weight it is hardly surprising that as many as 60 per cent of women with PCOS have 'disordered eating' patterns such as bulimia.

Cholesterol problems

A low level of the 'good' cholesterol – high density lipoprotein (HDL) – and an increased level of the 'bad' cholesterol – low density lipoprotein (LDL) – together with high triglyceride levels are seen in women with PCOS, particularly those who have insulin resistance.[12] This situation is associated with the risk of developing both heart disease and non-insulin-dependent (Type II) diabetes. Healthy eating and exercise can and are proven ways to help.

High blood pressure

Women with PCOS are four times more likely to suffer from high blood pressure than other people of the same age and weight. High blood pressure is an independent risk factor for heart disease.[13]

Non-insulin dependent diabetes

Research has shown that insulin resistance plays a significant role as both a cause and symptom of PCOS. A woman with PCOS is seven times more likely to develop diabetes during her lifetime than the rest of the population.[14]

Gestational diabetes

The increased incidence of hyperinsulinism and insulin resistance means that if you have PCOS you are likely to develop diabetes during pregnancy. This gestational diabetes can be associated with complications during pregnancy. After the pregnancy this type of diabetes commonly resolves, but there is an increased risk of it reappearing in later life.

Cardiovascular disease

Using the risk factors for cardiovascular disease which have been identified in women with PCOS, it is thought that they have a sevenfold increased risk of having a heart attack when compared to the general population.[15]

Endometrial cancer

We don't know if there is direct evidence of a link between PCOS and endometrial cancer, but we do know that this cancer is oestrogen-driven. If you have no periods, your womb lining doesn't shed, and this unshed, thicker lining can promote the cell changes linked to endometrial cancer.

Endometriosis

It is not uncommon to see both PCO/S and endometriosis in the same woman. Are the two conditions linked? No one really knows the answer at present. Endometriosis is a condition where tissue similar to the lining to the womb grows at other sites in the body outside the womb – commonly in the pelvis, on the ovaries and in the bowel, but also in rare cases on the lungs, eye, thighs and arms. We do know that this aberrant growth is oestrogen-dependent. Since many women with PCOS and irregular periods have raised oestrogen levels with little or no opposing progesterone, this may make the situation worse for women who also have endometriosis.

Ovarian cysts

A 1996 study reported an increased risk of ovarian cancer among women with PCOS in a population-based, case-controlled study involving 426 cancer patients and 4,081 controls.[16] The association was found to be stronger in those who had never used oral contraceptives. Many studies need to be done to verify these findings, and the link between PCOS and ovarian cancer is by no means established, but the relative protection offered by oral contraceptives needs to be taken into account when determining your choice of contraception.

But don't panic. Your body responds brilliantly to any help you give it to help prevent these health problems arising. Start now and you can reduce your risks.

First, change your food.

Eating well, managing stress, sleeping well and exercising regularly go a long way to keeping the doctor away and reducing the long-term health risks related to PCOS.

Many medical studies have shown that healthy eating can manage such conditions as diabetes. But paying attention to your diet can do more than manage health conditions like diabetes, it may even be able to *prevent* them occurring in the first place.

Diabetes

A 2001 Finnish study published in the *New England Journal of Medicine* suggests that a well-balanced diet can help to prevent diabetes in high-risk people. Researchers looked at over 500 overweight adults with impaired tolerance to glucose. The patients were divided into two groups, with the first group given advice from a nutritionist based on eating fewer fatty foods and more fruits and vegetables and cereals. They were also told about the benefits of exercise. The second group was not given this nutrition and exercise advice. After three years, 59 people in the second group developed diabetes, compared to only 27 in the group given eating and exercise guidelines.

Heart Protection

The British Heart Foundation dedicates itself to educating people about the dangers of high-fat, high-cholesterol diets. The message is clear: eating healthily can dramatically reduce your risk of a heart attack.

Increasing evidence has shown that eating five portions of fresh fruit and vegetables a day could cut the number of heart-disease and cancer deaths. In response to this evidence, doctors in one region of Britain have been prescribing vouchers which can be exchanged for fruit and vegetables. This experiment, taking place in the Wirral in the UK, aims to kick-start the changes in lifestyle and diet which can prevent illness.

Cancer

In 1997, the UK Government's Department of Health Committee on Medical Aspects of Food and Nutrition Policy took a rare step in publishing a report entitled *Nutritional Aspects of the Development of Cancer*. The World Health Organization (WHO) also acknowledges the fundamental role nutritional well-being plays in human development and the prevention of diseases like cancer and heart disease. WHO Director General Harlem Brundtland states, 'Nutrition is a cornerstone that affects and defines the health of all people rich and poor ... malnutrition makes us all vulnerable to disease.'

Recent research published in the *New England Journal of Medicine*, studying 45,000 pairs of twins, found that cancer is largely caused by diet and lifestyle choices rather than inherited risk.[17] Identical twins, who are genetically the same, were shown to have no more than a 15 per cent chance of developing the same cancer. This suggests that most cancers are at least 85 per cent due to environmental factors such as diet, lifestyle and exposure to toxic chemicals. This study found that choices about diet, smoking and exercise accounted for 58 to 82 per cent of the cancers studied.

Fertility Boost

Many fertility experts believe that a healthy diet can help you conceive and give birth to a healthy baby. It is among the first pieces of advice given to men and women thinking of starting a family. Research led by Leeds University Senior Registrar in Gynaecology, Dr Sara Matthews, on 215 UK women undergoing IVF treatment concluded that taking a daily multivitamin pill could boost a woman's fertility and double her chances of getting pregnant.

Healthy Children

It is also thought that a healthy diet and exercise programme can safeguard the future health of your children. Professor David Barker, Director of the UK's Medical Research Council Environmental Epidemiology Unit, warns that women who consistently eat poorly before conceiving could damage their baby's health and put their baby at an increased risk of cardiovascular disease later in life.

So eating right not only helps you deal with the day-to-day reality of living with PCOS, but can protect your health and the health of any children you have in the long term, by reducing the risk of future health problems.

If You Have Polycystic Ovaries (PCO)

Not all women with polycystic ovaries have any of the accompanying PCOS symptoms, so are described as having PCO and not PCOS.[18] For women with PCO, eating well now can help to prevent PCOS developing later.

If you are diagnosed with PCO, even though you may not feel unwell, environmental factors such as diet, stress and pollution can increase your risk of developing PCOS symptoms in the future. So you need to take extra care of yourself right now. A good diet is a sound investment for the future if you want to avoid PCOS.

GIVING YOUR MEDICATION A HELPING HAND

You may find that a change in diet is all you need to manage your symptoms, or you may decide to take some course of medicine, therapy or treatment once you are diagnosed with PCO/S. A good diet and nutritional programme is the essential foundation, in partnership with exercise for the management of PCOS. This type of programme works in conjunction with all kinds of medication for PCOS, from the Pill to fertility drugs, the diabetes drug Metformin and alternative therapies.

Dr Marilyn Glenville, one of the UK's leading nutritional therapists who treats women with PCOS in her London and Tunbridge Wells clinics, believes that a healthy diet will maximize your chances of health and fertility if you decide to take the Pill or use fertility drugs.

Belinda Barnes, director of Foresight (an organization which aims to improve a couple's fertility by giving advice about diet, nutritional supplementation, exercise and stress-management), says 'those that have IVF after having completed a Foresight nutritional program have a 65 per cent live birth success rate compared to the 14 per cent national average.'

Dr Ann Walker, a medical herbalist and research scientist based at the University of Reading's Hugh Sinclair Unit of Human Nutrition, explains that many herbalists and other complementary therapists will suggest beneficial changes to diet and lifestyle as the basis of good health. Walker believes that these are essential changes to make before herbalism, or any other medication, can come in and put the 'icing on the cake'. 'There is no point,' she says, 'in any medication coming in to suppress symptoms that are caused by a bad diet and unhealthy lifestyle. It is important to get the diet and lifestyle healthy first and then treat the remaining symptoms with medication. This often means that you need less medication, and what you do need works far more efficiently when the body is getting optimum nutrition in the first place.'

According to Gerard Conway, consultant gynaecologist at Middlesex Hospital, London, who has been working with women with PCOS to manage weight and improve symptoms using the diabetes drug Metformin, 'Metformin is not a magic bullet and can only work if diet and exercise plans are already in place.'

There have been several studies reporting good results with Metformin for weight loss. However, the goal is to use Metformin in conjunction with diet and exercise to lose weight, otherwise the effect of Metformin appears to wear off and doses need to increase. 'Weight gain often starts again unless there is a foundation of diet and exercise to start with which works in partnership with Metformin to produce better, more long-term results,' says Dr Conway.

EAT WELL AND PROSPER

What this book and the majority of PCOS experts believe is that diet and exercise are essential in managing PCOS regardless of which medicines, herbs, complements or fertility treatments you use on top of that.[19] Eating a healthy, well-balanced diet of fresh, whole foods in combination with moderate exercise is, in the words of Helen Mason, Senior Lecturer in Reproductive Endocrinology at St George's Hospital Medical School, London, 'the first-line treatment for women with PCOS'.

Living with PCOS is a major challenge. But as with any challenge, you can win and emerge from it looking and feeling great. Changing your eating habits may seem daunting right now, but the changes you need to make aren't complicated or unappetizing. All you need to do to improve the quality of your life right now, and in the years to come, is start making healthy food choices. It really is as simple as that.

Your PCOS Diet

Every food is a mix of different nutrients; the secret of a healthy diet for PCOS is to get the balance right. It also helps to know the reasons why you should be eating more of certain foods and less of others, so you can feel motivated to eat the right foods. This chapter will show you why you should eat the best foods for PCOS, and how you can go about doing this with a healthy eating plan.

Healthy eating can restore your blood-sugar and hormone balance, improve your energy levels, help you lose weight (if you need to) and address many PCOS symptoms. When the going gets tough, never lose sight of this.

YOUR DAILY FOOD BREAKDOWN

You are probably used to thinking of food in terms of calories, carbohydrates, proteins, fats, vitamins and minerals. Let's take a look at each of these in more detail.

A *calorie* is a unit of energy that is given off by a certain amount of food when it is burned or used for energy by your body.

Carbohydrates fuel your body with the energy it needs throughout the day and night. Next to fats, carbs are the most misunderstood part of our diet.

You need to understand their function in order to use them efficiently. Carbohydrates are divided into two groups: starches and sugars. Starches provide the complex carbohydrates which release a steady source of energy into your system. They satisfy your hunger far longer than the simple sugars found in sweets, cakes, biscuits and so on. Potatoes, brown pasta and wholemeal breads are typical sources of complex carbohydrates.

Proteins, found in meat, dairy products, legumes (peas, beans) and vegetables are important tissue-builders. While your body can use protein as an energy source, its prime function is to rebuild tissues and cells.

Fats, such as butter, margarine and oils, are another important energy source. Your body stores fat as an emergency supply for those times when you have used up your carbohydrate fuel.

Vitamins and *minerals* are essential to life. They contribute to good health by regulating the metabolism (energy you release from food) and working with enzymes – essential chemicals that are the foundation of all human bodily functions – to allow the activities that occur within your body to be carried out. They are called *micronutrients* because the body needs them in relatively small amounts compared with other nutrients like carbohydrates, proteins and fats. You can get all the vitamins and minerals you need for survival from fresh, healthful foods and sunlight, but you may need to boost with supplements to stay in the best of health for the long term.

10 STEPS TO A HEALTHIER YOU

In 1992 the US Department of Agriculture suggested that:

❈ 30–45 per cent of your calories should come from starchy (carbohydrate) foods – preferably whole grains such as wholewheat bread, brown rice, quinoa (a whole grain that cooks like white rice), wheat, oatmeal and rye

❈ 15–25 per cent from vegetables

❋ 10–15 per cent from fruit
❋ less than 10 per cent from meat and dairy products
❋ no more than 5 per cent from sugars and fats.

This is generally held to be a good model. Our diets would be far healthier if we stuck to these guidelines, but the truth is that the average Western diet consists of 37 per cent fat and 50 per cent refined carbohydrates and refined sugars. This diet is not healthy for most people, and can actually make the symptoms of PCOS worse.

The PCOS healthy eating plan has no gimmicks or secrets. You've seen that there is a link between nutrition and PCOS, and that changing the way you eat can ease symptoms now and protect your health in the future. Food is fuel. It helps your body function more smoothly. Scrimp on the quality and quantity of fuel and your body pays the price. That's true for everyone, but especially true if you have PCOS, because what you eat, when you eat and how much you eat directly affect your blood-sugar levels and hormone function.

So how do you eat right for PCOS? The principles are basically the same as for any healthy diet – sufficient complex carbohydrates, moderate amounts of protein, sufficient essential fats, a minimum of saturated fats and plenty of water. Each of the 10 easy-to-follow steps that follow focuses on one aspect of your diet.

1) Drink More Water

Drink plenty of water each day. Try to drink at least $1^1/_2$ litres/$2^3/_4$ pints (6 to 8 glasses) of fresh water each day.

Why?

We can exist without food for almost five weeks, but without water we can't last more than five days. Water gives us life and keeps us alive, yet we hardly give it a thought. Water is an essential – but often forgotten – nutrient. It's also absolutely crucial if you have PCOS.

Your body is made up of two-thirds water, so water intake and distribution is vital for hormonal function. You need to drink lots of water to keep your hormone systems working at their best. Water also helps to lubricate dehydrated and parched tissues, as well as aiding the body to eliminate waste by making fibre in your food swell and perform its function. It keeps your skin glowing and your cells working, and it delivers vitamins, minerals and other nutrients to your organs. For your liver to break down and excrete toxins and for your glands to secrete the correct balance of hormones, you need to drink plenty of pure water.

How?

If you don't drink enough you will start to feel dizzy, tired and could get headaches and stomach upsets. It's very important that you drink pure, clean (filtered, if necessary) water throughout the day, even if you don't feel thirsty. If you are feeling thirsty you are already dehydrated.

Should you have poor digestion, drink more water between meals and less during meals. When you're sick or under extra physical or emotional stress, drink more. If you're shorter or lighter than average you don't need to force yourself to drink as much as a taller, larger person. If it's hot or you are losing more fluids through perspiration, your fluid intake needs to be increased.

Don't forget that when you exercise your need will increase dramatically. Athletes in heavy training can use as much as 10 litres a day. Becoming dehydrated during exercise will have a major impact on your performance or ability to continue and get the maximum benefit. Even small losses of 2–3 per cent result in a 10 per cent reduction in strength.

Limit your tea, coffee and alcohol intake. This is because coffee, tea and alcohol raise blood-sugar levels, and therefore insulin levels. Water is the best drink for quenching thirst and hydrating the body to help prevent dry skin, sore eyes and wrinkles. Fresh fruit juice or diluted juice are suitable. Watch out for fruit juice 'drinks' posing as fresh fruit juice but which are really just expensive fakes. Try some of the better-quality squashes and cordials. There are also a wide number of very good herb and fruit 'teas' available (they aren't, strictly speaking, teas, but just use the name as they are infused with hot water).

Fruits and vegetables count towards your fluids because they consist of around 90 per cent water. They supply it in a form that is very easy for your body to use, at the same time as providing the body with a high percentage of vitamins and minerals.

One way to make sure you drink enough fluids is to fill a pitcher or a bottle with your targeted amount of water and drink it throughout the day. Take it with you in the car or to work, or keep it nearby when you're reading or doing other activities. If the container is empty by bedtime, you've achieved your goal.

2) Eat Five Portions of Fruit and Vegetables Each Day

Ideally, aim to eat at least three pieces of fruit and five portions of vegetables a day – that way you're bound to manage at least five. A vegetable portion is 1 to 2 cups of raw vegetables, 1 cup cooked. A fruit portion is 1 medium-sized apple, banana or orange.

Why?

For women with PCOS, all vegetables and most fruits are nutritional superstars. They are powerful sources of antioxidants, vitamins, minerals and phytochemicals (plant-based hormones). The vegetables highest in phytochemicals, such as cabbage, Brussels sprouts, cauliflower and broccoli, contain compounds which can help to lower androgen levels in the body (androgens are the male hormones responsible for PCOS symptoms such as acne and excess hair).

In addition to the newly discovered phytochemicals, orange, yellow and green fruits also provide the antioxidant beta-carotene, so helpful in boosting immune function. The dark green leafy vegetables such as broccoli are high in minerals that help make bones strong and can also calm the nervous system and help ease depression and anxiety. Fruit and vegetables also aid digestion because of their fibre content.

How?

Fruits are limited more than vegetables on the PCOS diet because many women have the tendency to eat them alone – particularly those like sugar-rich bananas and raisins which can give you an insulin rise if you don't eat them with proteins like a handful of nuts. All-fruit meals can upset your blood-sugar levels, creating that familiar peak followed by a slump in mood.

It may seem hard to fit in so many portions of fruit and vegetables, but vegetable soups and frozen and tinned fruits and vegetables all count. A very good way of boosting your intake is to invest in a juicer and make your own freshly-pressed juices such as apple and carrot, banana and apple, apple and celery, mango and pear or whatever mixture takes your fancy. For the best benefit, drink the juice as soon as you have made it, as contact with the air destroys vital vitamins and minerals. The downside of juicers is that they extract the pulp so you don't get the benefit of the fibre slowing down the release of sugar into your bloodstream. To get fibre, try using a blender to make smoothie-type drinks using berries and soft fruits such as pears, and soya milk or organic low-fat yogurt. You can also add in a teaspoon of Omega-3-rich oils such as hempseed or linseed (see page 40).

Eat whole fruits and whole vegetables wherever possible. These foods contain more fibre and generally have less of an effect on your blood-sugar than do refined, processed and juiced foods. A whole apple is better than apple juice, for instance, but fresh-pressed apple juice is better than juice from concentrate – and certainly better than nothing at all!

The way you prepare your fruits and vegetables will maximize their goodness. Heating, re-heating and storage often destroy nutrients, so try to eat as many as possible raw and fresh. Steaming or stir-frying are the best cooking methods to seal in the vital nutrients. If you do boil your vegetables, keep the water for a stock or a soup, as this is where all the nutrients will have gone.

Once a fruit or vegetable is picked or cut, it starts to lose nutrients. There is no telling how long fresh vegetables have lingered in the shop or warehouse (some are put in cold storage for as long as six months; others are picked long before they ripen to their most nutrient-rich state so that they can be flown across the world to another country before they go bad). Frozen vegetables are frozen immediately they are picked, so can sometimes be even better than fresh ones.

Ideally you should avoid peeling as much as possible, because vitamins often lie just beneath the skin of fruit and vegetables, but washing thoroughly or peeling is recommended for non-organic produce because of the potentially toxic effects of pesticides and fertilizers.

3) Eat Complex, Low-Glycemic Index (GI) Carbohydrates

Research is still ongoing about the optimal amount of carbohydrates for women with PCOS, but experts tend to agree that in general around 50 per cent of your total calories should come from carbohydrates, mostly in the complex form.

In addition to the carbohydrate in fruit and vegetables (see above) which counts towards this daily 50 per cent, try to eat four portions of wholegrains, such as brown rice, a day. One serving is one slice of bread or half a cup of cereal, cooked rice or pasta.

Why?

Carbohydrates are your body's prime energy source. They enable your body to use protein for growth and repair. Your body also uses carbohydrates, or starches, to make blood-sugar (glucose), which provides fuel used by the brain and muscles, including the heart.

In a balanced state your bloodstream contains about 2 teaspoons of glucose. The carbohydrates that you eat easily supply this amount of glucose, and it's all too easy to exceed the amount you need. The blood-sugar your body doesn't use as fuel is stored as body fat, under control of the hormone insulin. With your body's blood-sugar requirements so easily met, you don't want to be eating foods which rapidly turn into glucose and cause sharp rises in your blood-sugar level, followed by a sharp rise in your insulin level, followed by storage of excess blood-sugar as fat – in other words, the familiar PCOS symptoms of insulin resistance and weight gain.

We aren't telling you to eat fewer or more carbohydrates here. We're saying eat the right kind of carbohydrates. That is, complex and with a low GI (glycemic index). The key is to get enough blood-sugar over a sustained period of time, rather than a roller-coaster of highs and lows. Complex carbohydrates tend to take longer to convert into glucose, giving you sustained energy. Simple sugars tend to raise blood-sugar and worsen insulin resistance, exacerbating the hormone imbalances and fatigue typical in PCOS. Low-glycemic index foods also take longer to break down in the stomach and release their sugars. That's why you need to change the type of carbohydrate you eat rather than cutting them out altogether, and to make sure you combine them with protein – another way to help slow down the release of the sugars. Not eating carbohydrates is not healthy for women with PCOS in the long run. (At present, low-carb diets are fashionable. In Chapter 7 we'll discuss this in more detail.)

How?

Carbohydrates aren't just comfort foods, the sort of flour-based, stodgy cakes and breads we often turn to for a fix when we are feeling low. Fruits and vegetables are carbohydrates, too. So when we say 50 to 60 per cent of your daily intake comes from carbohydrates, this doesn't mean two-thirds of your diet should be bread and pasta. It means that you should eat more fruit and vegetables, while the rest of your intake should come from complex, low-GI carbs.

Because they break down into sugar slowly, complex carbohydrates like legumes, wholewheat bread and oats are generally better for you than simple carbohydrates found in sugary cereals, pies, cakes, biscuits and other processed food made from white sugar and/or white flour. Complex carbohydrates such as a fruit salad snack, a bowl of vegetable and lentil soup, or a handful of dried apricots and nuts, also provide more vitamins, minerals and dietary fibre than simple sugars.

In the glycemic index, carbohydrate foods are classified into three main groups according to how quickly they are turned into blood-sugar by the body. The higher a food appears on the index, the faster it induces insulin and therefore the greater its undesirability if you have PCOS. The lower a food's GI factor, the more slowly the food will convert into blood-sugar, promoting a weaker insulin response. Lowering blood-sugar levels will help balance your energy, reduce carbohydrate cravings, reduce insulin and testosterone levels and help you lose weight.

The Glycemic Index

The Glycemic Index was developed by David Jenkins in 1981 to express the rise of blood glucose (sugar) after eating a particular food.[1] The standard value of 100 is based on the rise seen with the digestion of glucose. The glycemic index ranges from about 20 for fructose and whole barley to about 95 to 98 for a baked potato. The glycemic index is used as a guideline for dietary recommendations for people with hypoglycemia or diabetes. Basically, a good starting point for people with PCOS (as for those with blood-sugar problems) is to avoid foods with high values and choose those with lower values. However, as we shall see, the glycemic index should not be the only dietary guideline on which to base your food choices.

Glycemic Index of Some Foods

Sugars	Fruits	Vegetables
Glucose 100	Apples 39	Beetroot 64
Maltose 105	Banana 62	Carrot, raw 31
Honey 75	Oranges 40	Carrot cooked, 36
Sucrose 60	Orange juice 46	Potato baked 98
Fructose 20	Raisins 64	Potato boiled 70

Most vegetables and many fruits have low GIs. The following have such low GIs that they can be eaten as often as you want, especially in their raw form:

❀ Apples
❀ Cabbage
❀ Celery
❀ Cherries
❀ Cucumber
❀ Lettuce
❀ Parsley
❀ Peaches
❀ Pears
❀ Plums
❀ Radishes
❀ Spinach
❀ Turnips
❀ Watercress

GIs of Other Foods

Grains	Legumes	Other foods
Bran cereal 51	Beans 31	Ice cream 36
Bread, white 69	Lentils 21	Milk 34
Bread, whole grain 72	Peas 39	Nuts 13
Corn 59		Sausages 28
Corn flakes 80		
Oatmeal 49		
Wholemeal pasta 45		
Rice 70		
Rice, puffed 95		

Make sure that at least half the grains you eat are whole grains. When whole wheat is milled into white flour, 25 nutrients are lost and only 5 added back. Other good choices include wholewheat pasta, wholewheat bread, oatmeal and basmati rice.

There are lots of easy ways you can increase your intake of complex carbohydrates:

Try wholegrain bread and cereals with some vegetable dips, fruit toppings or low-fat cottage cheese. Bear in mind that brown bread doesn't necessarily mean wholemeal. It could be white bread with added colourings. To be sure, read your food labels.

Try a different grain each week. Use oats, rye, barley, millet, rice, corn or buckwheat. Whole grains, like millet and quinoa, taste great and are simple to cook.

Add variety by eating rye bread or wholemeal scones with some low-fat spread and 100 per cent fruit jam.

Try some fruit bran or oatmeal cookies and muffins.

Fresh oatmeal porridge flavoured with chopped dried fruit is very satisfying.

Try a dish of brown rice with lean meat and vegetables in a curry sauce.

Eat Less Sugar

Try to limit your intake of sugary foods. Table sugar contains nothing but empty calories and goes right to your blood, where it raises blood-sugar and aggravates symptoms of PCOS. The US Department of Agriculture estimates that the average American consumes at least 64 pounds of sugar per year, and the UK is close behind. Most of the sugar doesn't come from the sugar bowl on the table but is hidden in our foods.

The USDA also found that people who eat diets high in sugar also consume fewer fruits and vegetables, and therefore get less nutrients. If you need another reason to lay off the sugar – apart from tooth and gum decay – research shows it can reduce the ability of white blood cells to fight infection, therefore making you more prone to colds and other illness.

Tips for Avoiding Sugar

– Look for breakfast cereals that contain no more than 5 grams of sugar per serving. The best bets are wholegrain cereals like granola/muesli, wheat flakes or hot cereal.

– Fat-free items often replace the fat with sugar, which makes them worse than their fatty counterparts for women with PCOS.

– You may think of sugar just in terms of white or brown, but there are many more forms: cane sugar, raw cane sugar, muscovado sugar, honey, treacle, syrup, molasses, dextrose, glucose, fructose, maltose, corn syrup, concentrated fruit juice, glucose syrup and other industrial sugars which are added to processed foods. They are all sugars and it is best to limit them.

– Reading labels to avoid these hidden sugars is one way of cutting down. Check the labels of your favourite sauces, spreads, cereals, biscuits and desserts for hidden sugars in the form of sucrose, glucose, dextrose, fructose, maltose, lactose, honey, corn syrup and so on.

– Limit your intake of sweets, biscuits, cakes, pies, doughnuts, pastries and other sweet baked goods. Eat fresh or dried fruit instead, or choose muffins or wholemeal fruit scones.

– Fruit drinks, beverages and cocktails are essentially noncarbonated soda pop. Most popular brands contain only 5 to 10 per cent juice. If you do choose them, go for high-juice brands, water them down with spring water or choose freshly pressed juice and add half water to it.

– Sugar substitutes aren't really a good idea for women with PCOS. Many metabolically-challenged people find these cause problems like headaches and stomach upsets. Best to avoid. Honey and syrups sound healthier but unfortunately they aren't. If your food really does need sweetening, a tiny bit of sugar is OK. Better still, add natural sweeteners like fruit juice or fresh fruits, or try the herbal alternative stevia, which is very sweet-tasting with no calories. You can buy this at your local health food store.

4) Eat a High-fibre Diet

Aim to eat 30 to 50 g of fibre daily. As a rough guide, an apple has around 2 g of fibre, and an orange 3 g. Eat your five portions of fruit and vegetables a day and you are halfway towards your fibre intake. You can get the rest of your fibre from complex carbohydrates. It's best to avoid large portions of bran, which act too fast and prevent you from absorbing vital nutrients.

Why?

Fibre is important if you have PCOS because it slows the conversion of carbohydrates into blood-sugar, thus helping maintain blood-sugar balance. It ensures that digestion is healthy, fat absorption is controlled, toxins are removed from the body, energy is released, stools are well formed and waste can pass through at a steady rate, preventing the build-up of hormones and toxins in the gut, from where they can be reabsorbed into the bloodstream. Moreover, fibre binds to excess cholesterol and oestrogens and escorts them from the body. An adequate fibre intake also ensures that you get that full-up feeling after you have eaten – great to help you stop snacking and overeating.

If you don't eat enough fibre, PCOS symptoms like weight gain, raised cholesterol, blood-sugar problems and excess testosterone and oestrogen are likely to get worse.

How?

You can get fibre in wholegrain cereals, nuts, seeds, fruits and vegetables or fibre supplements.

Only 30 to 50 g is needed; a diet rich in plant fibre easily supplies this. Drink plenty of fluid for the fibre to absorb to help it pass through your digestive system.

Fibre comes in two major sources, both essential for women with PCOS: *soluble* fibre, like oatmeal, dissolves in water and becomes soft and gel-like. This type of fibre slows down glucose absorption after a meal, keeping blood-sugar on an even keel. Soluble fibre also helps lower cholesterol. *Insoluble* fibre, like vegetables and bran, is dense and chewy, does not absorb water and stimulates movements in the intestines, thus preventing constipation. Insoluble fibre helps prevent diabetes, colon cancer and heart disease.

Research supports the idea of eating a high-fibre diet, especially for people with blood-sugar problems. Dr James Anderson at the University of Kentucky showed that diabetes control is greatly enhanced by eating a high-fibre diet. People with Type II diabetes in his study ate a diet composed of wholegrain cereal, vegetables and legumes in which not more than 25 per cent of the daily intake came from fat and 60 per cent came from carbohydrates. They also ate 50 g of fibre a day. After only a few weeks on the diet many people experienced better glucose control and were able to cut back on their medication.

Pectin, a type of fibre found in fruit and some vegetables, like carrots, along with fibre from legumes (such as beans and peas), oatmeal and barley, lowered the blood glucose response and insulin drive after a carbohydrate-rich meal. A study in the medical journal the *Lancet* showed that people with Type II diabetes who ate a cup and a half of legumes a day for six weeks had a 15 per cent reduction in fasting blood-glucose levels, as well as a 15 per cent reduction in their serum cholesterol levels.

Another reason to make fibre-rich fruits and vegetables and wholegrains the foundation stones of your diet: you get your healthy low-GI complex carbs and fibre all in one go.

If you aren't used to a high-fibre diet, you need to introduce more fibre slowly to give your bowels time to adapt. Don't be surprised if your stools look bulkier the more fibre you eat.

After two years of skipping periods, starting to get excess facial hair and being so overweight, I decided I had to go to the doctor. She saw my facial hair and I told her I didn't have periods any more and she said she thought I may have PCOS. I was like 'Huh?!?' She told me I was insulin resistant and sent me to a diabetes centre to learn about diet. Basic stuff really about eating little and often, making sure you get all your nutrients, increasing your fibre intake and watching that you don't eat foods which trigger blood-sugar problems. I made some changes to my diet and started a gentle walking programme. The first week or so I nearly gave up. I thought something was wrong. I needed the restroom several times a day, but the dietician told me that this was just my digestive system adjusting and it would clear up soon. She was right. It did.

When I went back to the doctor after 6 weeks I knew I had lost some weight and I was feeling better, but I never suspected how good the news would be. In 6 weeks I had lost 35 pounds! And six months later not only had I continued to lose weight, reaching my target weight, but my periods had returned. Today I'm doing fine. I still get the occasional blip if I don't take care of myself, but I know what to do. I sometimes feel sorry for myself that I have to be so disciplined, but then I remind myself of how good it feels to be healthy and not be ashamed of the way I look.
Linda, 39

5) Eat Good-quality Protein with Every Meal

Eat two to five portions of protein each day, which should include some vegetable sources such as beans, lentils and tofu. Include protein such as dairy products, lean meat (chicken, turkey) eggs, tofu, soya milk, pulses (beans, lentils – also an excellent source of fibre), nuts and/or seeds with every meal. One portion is about 3 oz of cooked meat or fish (which is about the size of a deck of cards), one egg or half a cup of beans.

Why?

Protein helps maintain blood-sugar balance and gives your body an even supply of the amino acids it needs to build and repair cells and manufacture hormones and brain chemicals. Since your body can't store amino acids, as it does carbohydrates and fat, you need a constant supply of them. That's why you need to eat some high-quality protein with every meal.

The amino acids are called 'the building blocks of life' because the body uses them to rebuild and repair its tissues and organs. If water were removed from your body, more than half of its dry weight would be protein. Your skin, hair, nails, muscles, metabolic enzymes, neurotransmitters and, most importantly for PCOS, your hormones are all composed of protein.

Proteins perform many life-enhancing functions inside our bodies. It's also worth remembering that proteins, like fats, have a stabilizing effect on blood-sugar, producing steady, long-term energy instead of a short burst followed by a quick let-down. Eating complete proteins in the form of fish, poultry, lean meat, low-fat cottage cheese, eggs, soy and whey stimulates the production of the pancreatic hormone glucagon. Glucagon performs the opposite role to insulin: it helps to mobilize stored fat for use as a fuel source, thus keeping insulin levels lower.

And finally, without a reasonable amount of protein to rebuild your muscles it is not possible to increase your muscle mass. The more muscle mass you have, the faster your metabolic rate, because muscles burn more calories, even when you don't do any exercise, than any other tissue. The faster your metabolic rate, the easier it is for you to lose weight and manage your symptoms.

How?

The recommended daily allowance (RDA) of protein for sedentary individuals is 0.75 g per kilogram of body weight. However, for those who are trying to get fit and develop their muscles, this may not be enough. Everyone's individual requirement will vary – a dietician can advise you on this.

Good sources of protein which are low in unhealthy fats include chicken, turkey breast and oily fish. Try to eat plain, live yogurt – preferably daily (if you have a cow's milk allergy, try other sources – soya, goat's milk, sheep's milk) – as it contains beneficial bacteria that populate the gut and support your digestion.

A Word about Soy

Soy protein in the form of tofu (bean curd, usually sold in blocks) and soy milk are vegetarian protein sources. However, some women find that soy foods produce allergic reactions such as a rapid heart rate and rashes. If you are sensitive to soy you can derive the benefits from supplements or pills rather than the food itself. Excess soy can also upset your body's mineral balance, leading to problems like panic attacks and hair loss. So don't use soy as your only source of protein. Once again, moderation is key.

Excess protein intake is not wise if you have PCOS. If you fill up on proteins you have less room for nutrient-rich foods that can help balance blood-sugar levels. If you do eat animal protein, limit your intake to 2 or 3 oz per meal – a serving size no bigger than the palm of your hand. Where possible eat organic animal foods to avoid consuming the growth hormones and antibiotics with which many non-organic animals are routinely treated.

A sensible balance is two portions of carbohydrate to every one portion of protein, and no less than one portion of carbs to one portion of protein. One portion of protein equals 3 oz of cooked, lean meat or fish, half a cup of baked beans, 3 oz of hard cheese, 2 eggs or three-quarters of a cup of cottage cheese. To avoid a large intake of animal protein and an increase in saturated fat, it is possible to eat vegetarian sources of protein.

Try to include a range of protein in the form of low-fat cottage cheese, ricotta cheeses, quark cheese, lean red meat, poultry, seafood, fish and egg whites. Other sources of proteins are soybeans, split peas, kidney beans, peas, wheatgerm, lima beans, black-eyed peas, lentils, black beans, spirulina and grains such as quinoa.

Proteins and fats are digested more slowly than carbohydrates and will slow down the entry of sugar into your blood. Dried beans and peas can lower the effect of other carbohydrate-rich foods on your blood-sugar. When eaten alone, legumes don't raise blood-sugar very much even though they contain carbohydrate, but when eaten together with other carbohydrate-rich foods they can actually lower the effect these foods have on your bloodstream. For example, when you eat pinto beans with rice, the beans reduce the effect of the rice on blood-sugar. Similarly, if you really want to eat that cake, make sure you eat it as part of a meal that includes beans.

Ideally your protein intake should be split throughout the day so that at every meal you take in some protein along with carbohydrates from wholegrains, vegetables and fruits. This will help reduce your insulin production levels in response to the amount of carbohydrate eaten. But if you do find it hard to digest food or have irritable bowel syndrome (IBS) or digestive problems, food combining (taking proteins and carbs at separate meals) can often help to ease the problem until you can work up to a diet where you can mix the two (see page 174).

For Vegetarians and Vegans

When you look at the diets of most vegetarians, protein intake tends to be small. If you are a vegetarian it is very important that you get complete proteins in your meal. Below are some suggestions to help you do this.

– If you are the only vegetarian in your household, make sure you substitute pulses, beans, wholegrain cereals, dairy products, tofu products or quorn instead of just leaving the meat part out of the meal.
– Choose cereals fortified with vitamins, especially B_{12}. (And don't forget, Marmite is a good source of this vitamin.)
– Try to eat a large portion of dark green leafy vegetables every day, and half to three-quarters of a pint of semi-skimmed milk a day to ensure your calcium intake. If you are lactose intolerant you can get your calcium in soya yogurts and milks or nut milks.

– Eat dried fruits, pulses, green vegetables and whole grains for fibre and iron. Cocoa powder and dark chocolate are good sources of iron, too.
– Eat at last 30 g of pulses, nuts and seeds every day for protein and EFAs.
– Eat at least one serving of low-fat cheese or cottage cheese a day for protein and calcium – or a soya pattie or tofu portion.
– Eat a total of three to four eggs a week.
– Choose margarine or butter fortified with vitamin D and E in a vegetarian spread. You can get vitamin D from sunlight as well, and vitamin E from nuts and seeds.

If you are a vegan, the risk of nutritional deficiencies is higher. You need to seek expert advice from a doctor or nutritionist. The Vegan Society has lots of useful information (see Chapter 12).

Your biggest concern as a vegan is to ensure you get adequate amounts of protein and vitamin B_{12}. The American Diabetic Association states that soy protein has been shown to be nutritionally equivalent to animal protein. Nuts, seeds, grains, pulses and vegetables are other good sources of protein. Yeast extracts used as food flavourings are often high in B_{12}; if you are a vegan, eat these foods regularly, together with other products such as cereals, with a guaranteed vitamin B_{12} content. You can also take a B-complex vitamin supplement which includes B_{12}.

6) Make Sure You Get Enough Essential Fatty Acids (EFAs)

As a guideline, calories from fats should contribute 20 to 25 per cent of your total calories in your diet. You should try to obtain as little fat as possible from the saturated, animal fats or transfatty acids found in many commercial foods, and as much as possible in the form of essential fatty acids (EFAs) such as the Omega-3 and Omega-6 fatty acids.

Why?

Many conditions, including PCOS, are associated with the metabolism of fatty acids. Our bodies need essential fats to regulate hormone function and strengthen cell walls. Some of the health benefits of special concern to women with PCOS include: improvement in skin, hair and nails, and regular periods. What's more, high-quality dietary fat slows down the entry of carbohydrates to the system, thus keeping insulin levels lower, and satisfies your hunger. In fact, dietary fat is the best blood-sugar stabilizer. And stable blood-sugar means less depression, greater mental focus and improvement of PCOS symptoms.

Without sufficient quantities of Omega-3 and Omega-6 fatty acids, your body cannot manufacture many important substances including ovarian and stress hormones. If you are eating a very low-fat diet you won't be getting enough of these EFAs, and this can affect your menstrual cycle.

How?

Nuts, seeds, olive oil, avocado, flaxseed oil and oily fish (mackerel, salmon, herrings and sardines) are rich in essential fatty acids. Aim to eat fish at least twice a week, and nuts and seeds (flax, sunflower, pumpkin, hemp, sesame, almonds, cashews, walnuts) daily, maybe as a snack between meals, take flax oil by the tablespoon or in salad dressings, add hempseed oil to smoothies, or use sesame oil with stir-fries.

Omega-3 fatty acids are far less common than Omega-6 fatty acids in our modern diets. Omega-3 fatty acids are found in the oils of cold-water fish as well as in some seeds (including hemp seeds and pumpkin seeds) and in walnuts. Omega-6 fatty acids are in many foods, especially nuts, seeds, vegetable oils (such as sunflower, soy, walnut, sesame, olive, coconut and peanut oil) and legumes. The two types of fat are not interchangeable; you need to consume both and keep them balanced.

If you don't eat fish, flaxseed oil or flax seeds (also known as linseeds) are excellent sources of Omega-3: **7 grams** of flaxseed oil are equivalent to 1 gram of fish oil. Try a daily dose of 3 heaped teaspoons of cold-pressed flaxseed oil or three tablespoons of ground flax seed. Hempseed, pumpkin seed or soybean oil are also good sources. Use only cold-pressed vegetable oils; the bottle should say 'unrefined', 'unhydrated' or 'cold-pressed'. Alternatively, grind 1 tablespoon of seeds and mix it into cereals or sprinkle over salads. Sea vegetables (edible seaweed, kelp, etc.) and green leafy vegetables are also good sources.

It's best to avoid refined and processed foods, as they contain substances which can block the absorption of EFAs, and limit your intake of excess fatty foods from animal sources such as lamb and pork, high-fat cheeses and cream. Animal fats contain a substance that encourages blood-clotting and inflammation – thus they can exacerbate eczema or other inflammatory conditions. Game is less fatty, as are white meats, poultry and fish. Steer clear of factory-farmed poultry, which often contains hormones and antibiotics that can upset your hormonal, immune and digestive systems.

You don't need to avoid animal fat completely, simply keep it to a minimum, but do avoid vegetable oils in the form of the fried, oxidized or hydrogenated fats found in margarine, vegetable shortenings and fast-food french fries. The 'transfatty acids' found in many processed foods, margarines, baked goods and takeaway chips, as well as cereals, peanut butter, mayonnaise and snack foods, should be avoided because they can increase the risk of diabetes, according to research by the *New England Journal of Medicine*. These can also be called hydrogenated fats or oils on labels.

To sum up: Reducing the amount of red meat you eat in your diet to three meals or fewer a week, switching to extra-virgin olive oil, increasing your intake of oily fish to three portions a week, eating more vegetarian meals and snacking sensibly on mixed nuts and seeds during the day rather than crisps or sweets are all easy ways to ensure correct and healthy fat consumption.

7) Stock Up on Phytonutrients

Phytonutrients are the hidden health-givers in our food. Ensure that you include them in your diet on a daily basis.

Why?

Phytonutrients or phytochemicals are health-supporting substances that occur naturally in plants and give them colour, flavour and natural disease resistance. You can survive without phytonutrients, but you won't feel or look very good. Hundreds of scientific studies support the theory that these plant compounds with impossible-to-pronounce Latin names may be our life-savers, by affecting our health as significantly as vitamins and minerals, offering natural protection against all kinds of disorders and reducing the risk of diabetes, heart disease and memory loss.

As they are not stored in your body, you need to eat foods rich in phytochemicals on a regular basis to benefit your heart, skin, hair and mental and reproductive health.

If you have PCOS, ensure that you stock up on phytonutrients every day.

How?

It's quite simple, really. Just make sure you meet your daily fruit and vegetable food requirements. Plant-based foods are brimming with phytonutrients. The best strategy is to include a wide variety of colourful fruits and vegetables in your diet on a daily basis. Variety is the key. Eating a few apples and a banana a day is OK, but not as good as being more adventurous. Research shows that those who eat a diet with a varied mix of vegetables have a 20 per cent lower risk of colon cancer than those whose intake is less varied. A useful trick is to think about the colours of the rainbow when you choose your fruits and vegetables. A good selection of colours will mean that you get a good selection of phytonutrients. So aim for multicoloured meals – check orange, yellow, red, purple and green are all present by choosing foods such as mangoes, blackberries, cabbage, peppers, carrots, etc. The deeper the colour, the more phytochemicals are present.

The main groups of phytochemicals include: flavonoids (these give grapefruit its tartness and cherries their blush, and reduce the risk of heart disease and stroke); phytoestrogens (in soya, tofu, pulses and sprouts – they reduce the risk of breast cancer and improve bone strength); carotenoids (they give orange and green fruit and veg their colour and protect against heart disease, cancer and Alzheimer's disease.)

You'll Like This

It's only since the advent of phytochemical research that red wine has been found to be good for you (it's packed with a phytochemical called reseveratrol). Also, 40 g of chocolate has a similar phytochemical content to a glass of red wine. It also has the undesirable type of fat and sugar, so has some disadvantages, but proves once again that everything can be good in moderation. Tea, especially green tea, is a rich source of phytochemicals. Four cups of green tea gives you optimal amounts of epicatechin, which has antioxidant, antibacterial, antiviral, anticancer and immune-enhancing properties. If you don't like green tea, look for black tea blends with green tea added.

Vegetables highest in phytochemicals are cabbage, Brussels sprouts, cauliflower, broccoli and other green leafy vegetables. Fruits high in phytochemicals include tomatoes, cranberries and blueberries. The 30 best sources of phytochemicals identified to date are:

apples	cherries	pineapples
aubergines	chillies	red peppers
avocados	garlic	red wine
bananas	grapefruit	rye
barley	green tea	sesame seeds
bean sprouts	leeks	soya (including tofu)
berries	milk	spinach
broccoli	oats	tomatoes

carrots	oranges	walnuts
celery	parsley	whole wheat

8) Eating to Reduce Cholesterol

Include foods in your diet such as oats, which have been proved especially useful in reducing cholesterol levels.

Why?

Cholesterol is a fatty, wax-like substance produced by stress, biochemical and hormonal reactions and food, primarily in your liver but also in your intestines and other cells within your body.

Cholesterol isn't all bad news. It plays an essential role in bodily processes including the production of sex hormones such as oestrogen and progesterone. Cholesterol, as with other blood fats, only creates a problem when you have too much of it. Too much cholesterol can promote the production of fatty plaque which can clog up your arteries. If this happens, the blood flow is interrupted and this could lead to a heart attack or stroke. Blocked arteries also cause circulation problems, numbness and pain in your feet and hands.

Nutritionally you need to keep the risk of fatty plaque-blockage as low as possible. You can do this by eating foods which stimulate the production of 'good' cholesterol (high-density lipoprotein – HDL) and avoiding foods which stimulate 'bad' cholesterol. (Low-density lipoprotein – LDL). HDL carries excess amounts of LDL back to your intestines where it is excreted. It doesn't matter how much HDL you have in your blood – the thing to watch out for is raised LDL.

You can encourage your body to excrete LDL by taking in more beneficial foods. In addition, you can ensure that your diet contains plenty of the nutrients that prevent LDL from forming deposits in your blood vessels.

The Pill

It is important to point out that the contraceptive pill, the most common medicine for PCOS, lowers HDL and increases LDL levels. If you have PCOS and have been or are on the contraceptive pill, it is crucial that you check your LDL levels regularly with your doctor and pay attention to your diet.

Controlling cholesterol is vital for everyone, and especially for women with PCOS in order to protect against heart disease, especially as low levels of good cholesterol and increased levels of bad cholesterol are seen in women with PCOS, particularly those with insulin problems. This situation is associated with the risk of developing heart disease and diabetes.[2] It is estimated that women with PCOS have a 7-fold increased risk of having a heart attack when compared to the general population.[3]

How?

Regular exercise is one of the best ways to reduce cholesterol (see Chapter 7), but certain foods can stimulate your body to produce HDL. Garlic has a substance that has this effect, as do oily fish such as herrings, mackerel, sardines, tuna and salmon. Oily fish contains Omega-3, which can help your body carry more LDL to the intestines to be excreted. Other foods which are thought to lower cholesterol include fresh fruit, vegetables and olive oil. Kidney beans and other legumes such as chickpeas, as well as soy-based foods are also thought to lower the risk of raised LDL levels.

Aim to have at least two or three meals containing garlic/oily fish a week. Why not try freshly grilled sardines, herrings, tuna steaks or salmon, or make fish soups and garlic dips? Add garlic to pasta sauces and stir-fries, or you can take a daily supplement.

Fresh garlic (which is in the shops for a couple of months every year) is the most potent, but during the rest of the year the older garlic is fine. If you find the smell of garlic a little anti-social, try chewing fresh parsley or coffee beans after you've eaten it to reduce the potency of the smell, or you can take an odour-controlled supplement.

Make sure you eat enough fibre in your diet. Fibre produces substances which help your body excrete more LDL. Fibre also prevents large amounts of fat being absorbed, so that more LDL is kept bound within the gut and excreted. Eating vegetables (including beans and lentils), fruits and whole grains, bread, pasta and rice every day really helps to bring your blood fat profile within the ideal range.

Oats are rich in a particular fibre that has proved especially useful in reducing cholesterol levels. Try to include oats in your meals at least once or twice a week – as oatcakes, flapjacks, porridge oatmeal (from healthfood shops) or in fruit crumbles.

In addition to watching your saturated fat intake, eating plenty of fruits and vegetables will also have a beneficial effect – and don't forget the very pleasant idea of drinking a glass of red wine (ideally, organic) every day. Red wine contains antioxidants which can help reduce cholesterol.

If you follow the other healthy eating guidelines in this chapter for fibre, EFAs, complex carbs and fruits and vegetables, you will already be eating a diet that can lower your risk of high LDL levels. As you can see, all these eating guidelines work towards the same goal – improving your health and your PCOS symptoms.

9) Spice Up Your Life

Instead of salt, try herbs, spices, lemon juice or root ginger to flavour your food.

Why?

Salt causes fluid retention and can raise blood pressure. Women with PCOS are four times more likely to suffer from high blood pressure than age- and weight-matched controls.[4]

Blood pressure is the force exerted by the blood on the inner walls of the blood vessels. A blood-pressure measurement is expressed as one number over another, e.g. 120/80. The upper (systolic) value reflects the force with which the heart pumps blood around the body, while the other (diastolic) value is the pressure in the blood vessels when they are relaxed. Normal blood pressure readings for women are in the region of 120/80. The bottom figure is the one to watch in establishing whether or not you have hypertension – the medical name for high blood pressure. Anything over 90 is considered hypertensive.

If hypertension is ignored, it can lead to an increased risk of heart disease, strokes or kidney problems. Sometimes drugs are needed to lower blood pressure, but most of the time blood pressure can be controlled through nutrition and lifestyle changes.

How?

To reduce your risk of high blood pressure you should ensure that you eat a healthy diet according to the guidelines given in this chapter. A healthy diet can provide your body with all that it needs to reduce your blood pressure. Especially watch your cholesterol level, eat lots of fruit and vegetables, sufficient essential fatty acids and foods high in calcium (such as low-fat yogurt or cheese). Calcium has been shown to be helpful in correcting high blood pressure, so you should try to include some low-fat dairy products in your diet. If you don't like or have an allergy or intolerance to dairy products, other sources of calcium include white bread, spinach and sesame seeds.

Finally, limit your intake of salt. Watching the amount of salty foods you eat can reduce blood pressure. Salt (sodium chloride) is found naturally in small amounts in many foods, especially manufactured ones, both as a preservative and flavour-enhancer. You can't avoid salt altogether but you can take steps to reduce your sodium intake.

Bear in mind that many food labels list salt as 'sodium' or 'sodium chloride'. Some foods claim to be 'reduced salt' or 'low salt' and so on, but this can be confusing when the label talks in terms of sodium. The sodium content of food must be shown, but not all manufacturers and retailers add a salt equivalent. To find out how much salt is in the food, multiply the sodium content figure by 2.5. Aim for less than 5 g of salt a day.

Try to get out of the habit of adding unnecessary salt in cooking. Taste before you add any.

The following foods are very high in salt and should be avoided, if possible:

✿ table/cooking salt
✿ cured and smoked meats
✿ smoked and pickled fish
✿ canned meats
✿ salted butter and margarine/spreads (unless low-salt)
✿ savoury crackers and other snacks
✿ salted nuts
✿ some sweet biscuits
✿ baked beans and some canned vegetables (look for those with no added salt or sugar)
✿ olives in brine
✿ sauces, ketchup, brown sauce, soy sauce
✿ stock cubes (look for salt-free or low-salt varieties in healthstores)
✿ canned fish in brine

Moderate- to Low-salt Foods
✿ fresh fruit and vegetables
✿ wholemeal flour and pasta
✿ brown rice
✿ breakfast cereals without added salt, like shredded wheat, puffed rice
✿ unsalted butter and low-salt spreads
✿ nuts
✿ dried fruits
✿ pulses

✿ oatmeal and oats
✿ poultry
✿ game
✿ meat
✿ eggs

Instead of salty preserved meats, choose the fresh alternative such as fresh salmon and lean beef.

Bread, hard cheese, cereals, oily fish (e.g. kippers, smoked mackerel and canned fish, especially in brine) are highly salted foods but they should not be avoided (unless on doctor's orders) as they provide other important and protective nutrients.

Instead of salt, experiment with herbs and spices or other alternatives. Basil, chervil, chives, dill, fennel and garlic work well with salads. Thyme, tarragon and parsley can really enhance the flavour of meat, fish, vegetables and potatoes. Wine is a wonderful flavour-enhancer. When it is boiled the alcohol evaporates, leaving behind the aromatic essence of the wine. Mustard really brings out the flavour of cheese. Have fun experimenting with spices or alternatives to salt until you find those you like best.

You will gradually be able to adjust to a less salty diet and learn to appreciate the more subtle flavours that were once hidden by the overpowering taste of salt.

10) Get Snacking

Start the day with a good breakfast, have a mid-morning snack, followed by lunch, a mid-afternoon snack and then supper.

Why?

The typical way many of us find ourselves eating is a small or non-existent breakfast followed by a light snack at lunch and then a big evening meal. Sometimes people don't eat at all until their evening meal, which can be as late as 8.30 p.m. Stacking your calories like this isn't a very good idea, especially if you have PCOS.

First of all, you are telling your body that once you get up in the morning you are fasting. In the fasted state your body will do its best to hold on to every last calorie, as it is not sure when it will get the next one. Your body achieves this very effectively by reducing your metabolic rate. Not only this, but in the fasted state, because of your brain's absolute requirement for glucose, you begin to break down your own muscle to provide the necessary glucose.

You can't convert fat into glucose. The net effect is a loss in muscle mass and reduction in your metabolic rate. Then when you do eat in the evening, your body is now set up to store as much fat as possible. After eating you often go to bed, so your body has little time to use any of the calories that you have just consumed.

Missing breakfast and fasting during the day isn't a good idea because it encourages weight gain, sends your body confusing signals and deprives your body and your mind of the energy they need to function optimally. If you have PCOS and are worried about weight gain, you aren't doing yourself any favours with such an uneven food intake during the day.

How?

Start the day with breakfast, have a mid-morning snack, followed by lunch, afternoon tea, then supper. All you need to get right is *what* to eat at each of these meal times. Obviously they do not need to be large meals, but should combine complex, low-GI carbohydrates with small amounts of protein.

Try to eat most of your calories earlier in the day. This would avoid being in 'fast mode' during the day and allow some of the calories to be burned off during the day's activities.

Breakfast is often the meal that is completely ignored, but it's the most important one. It kick-starts your metabolism, gives you energy and sets you up for the day. You may not feel like eating two minutes after you have jumped out of bed, so try and give yourself a little time to wake up before eating. Preparing something for later in the day such as a few snacks will start your digestive system working. Then eat some breakfast.

It's a good idea to cook a little extra the night before so that you have snacks for the rest of the day to take to work or eat at home. An extra chicken breast, piece of salmon or pot of reduced-fat hummus together with some vegetable sticks such as carrots, celery and cucumber are simple and will work wonders at 11 a.m. and 3 p.m. when you start to wilt, as would some fresh or dried fruit and a handful of walnuts, almonds or sunflower seeds.

When I was diagnosed with PCOS my doctor told me that it would be harder for me to lose weight, and suggested regular exercise. I'd never been that health-conscious but wanted to lose the weight, so I enrolled in a gym and started classes a few times a week. I also made sure I was eating healthily. After six months nothing had happened – in fact, I had gained 5 pounds. I felt as if I was destined to be overweight.

In frustration I contacted a dietician who had experience helping women with PCOS. She asked me to tell her what I was actually eating, and she agreed that I wasn't eating too much and that my food choices were sound. She said that the problem was I was skipping breakfast, not eating much at lunchtime and eating my main meal at night. She told me that the answer wasn't a diet but to move towards a more metabolically-sound eating pattern. This meant six meals a day to keep my metabolic rate high so more food is burned off. Basically I was to eat the same amount of food, but in a different order. It seemed like her advice was far too generous – and how was I going to cope with eating breakfast, something I hadn't done in years? Within weeks of changing my eating schedule, though, I was pounds lighter. All those years of

skipping breakfast because I thought it would help me lose weight were actually making me gain it! How wrong can you be?
Rebecca, 27

Healthy Snacks
- ❀ glass of fresh-pressed (not from concentrate) fruit juice
- ❀ 4 fresh apricots
- ❀ 3 fresh dates
- ❀ 1 dried date
- ❀ 1 plum
- ❀ 1 pear
- ❀ 1 apple
- ❀ 1 rice cake
- ❀ 1 jaffa cake
- ❀ 1 fig roll
- ❀ 1 small pain au raisin
- ❀ 1 low-fat granola/muesli bar
- ❀ 1 low-fat scone/muffin/flapjack
- ❀ 2 breadsticks with vegetable dips
- ❀ handful of nuts and seeds
- ❀ low-fat yogurt and a cracker
- ❀ low-fat cottage cheese and a cracker
- ❀ tuna on toast
- ❀ 2 dark rye Ryvita with Marmite
- ❀ celery and carrot sticks
- ❀ low-fat cottage cheese topped with apple sauce and walnuts
- ❀ natural sugar-free wholegrain muffins
- ❀ freshly made unsalted popcorn
- ❀ rice cakes topped with nut butter
- ❀ watermelon, fresh fruit or frozen fruit popsicles
- ❀ unsweetened low-fat yogurt topped with granola/muesli or nuts and fresh fruit

Eating Out

Healthy eating doesn't mean that you can't eat out anymore. You just need to pay a little more attention to what you are ordering. Here are some helpful tips:

❀ Stay away from the bread basket.

❀ Drink water or fruit juice instead of fizzy, sugar-loaded drinks.

❀ Try vegetable soup for starters.

❀ Ask for vegetables instead of chips/fries.

❀ Have a side salad with your main course.

❀ Go for tomato- or wine-based sauces rather than cheesy, buttery sauces.

❀ Ask for salad dressings (olive oil, vinegar) on the side so you can dress it yourself.

❀ Have a fruit-based dessert.

❀ Don't be afraid to ask for food not on the menu, such as fruit salad.

❀ At Chinese or Indian restaurants, choose plain, boiled rice rather than fried. Healthier Indian food comes from the tandoor oven which cooks chicken tandoori, tikka and sekh kebab dishes. Look out for ghee and butter in sauces.

❀ Choose clear soups rather than thickened or 'cream of' ones.

❀ Charcoal-grilled or roasted fish and kebabs are better than fried.

❀ Look for salads and simple stuffed vegetable dishes if you enjoy Mediterranean food. Fresh fish dishes are also a good bet.

❀ At Mexican restaurants, bypass the tortilla chips and cheese and stick to the salsa, fresh and steamed vegetables and grilled meats.

❀ Don't be afraid to ask for an ingredient to be left out of a dish – for example freshly-made pizza without the cheese, tortilla chips without sour cream, salad without the dressing.

❀ If you are eating out later than usual, eat a balanced snack when you would normally have eaten dinner. You won't be as hungry when you arrive at the restaurant. If your plate arrives very full, eat only half and ask the waiter to put the rest in a doggy bag and have it for lunch the next day.

'AT A GLANCE' TABLES OF FOODS RICH IN NUTRIENTS

Protein	EFAs	Complex and low GI carb	Phytonutrients	Fibre
Low-fat cottage cheese	Nuts	Wholegrain bread	Soya	Oats
Lean red meat	Seeds	Oats	Chickpeas (garbanzo beans)	Apples
Fish	Pumpkin seeds	Oatbran	Lentils	Wholegrain bread, pasta, etc.
Chicken	Walnuts	Dried fruits	Garlic	Squash
Soy	Linseed (flaxseed) oil	Basmati or parboiled rice	Celery	Carrots
Egg whites	Broccoli	Green and brown lentils	Seeds	Most fruits and vegetables
Soybeans	Tuna	Soybeans	Sesame seeds	
Split peas	Mackerel	Baked beans	Sunflower seeds	
Kidney beans	Sardines	Wholegrain pasta	Rice	
Peas	Salmon	Apples	Oats	
Wheat germ		Oranges	Apples	
Lima beans (butter beans)		Peaches	Cherries	
Black eyed peas		Plums	Plums	
Lentils			Carrots	
			Alfalfa	
			Mung	
			Beansprouts	

MAKING YOUR EATING PLAN A SUCCESS

The healthy diet guidelines recommended in this chapter centre around carbohydrates with low GIs, phytochemical-rich fruits and vegetables, protective fats and quality protein to help balance blood-sugar levels, ease carbohydrate cravings and improve digestion, absorption and elimination – all of which are crucial for proper hormonal balance.

Stable blood-sugar levels can prevent many PCOS symptoms and encourage weight loss. What's more, a balanced blood chemistry enables you to control cravings for unhealthy food. As time goes on and you make gradual improvements, you will begin to see that you don't have to rely on will-power alone to eat right. Once you start eating more healthily, your appetite adjusts and certain foods, which you know can trigger symptoms, just don't seem so tempting any more.

With all the benefits that a healthy diet can offer for PCOS, it can be tempting to rush straight in and make dramatic changes. But as you try to incorporate these 10 steps into your life, remember that changing the way you eat takes time. Start by making changes little by little to what and when you eat, and as each week passes you will start to notice gradual improvements in your symptoms and the way you look and feel. In time you won't just be surviving anymore – you'll be flourishing!

Try not to set yourself up for failure, and remember the 80/20 rule. You can't eat healthily 100 per cent of the time. The occasional treat – a bar of chocolate, a sweet pastry or a bag of chips – doesn't mean that you have failed. It is the excesses that are potentially dangerous. It's important that you enjoy your food and allow yourself the occasional indulgence. So no food is off-limits.

There are lots of diets out there. If you have PCOS and want to lose weight or boost your energy levels, it's best to avoid fad diets and take the smart route by following the healthy diet guidelines outlined in this chapter, together with (if necessary) the weight-loss guidelines in Chapter 7.

I've heard all about the low-carb diet, and how it is supposed to help women with PCOS, but weren't we told for years to cut down on protein and fat? I know lots of women who lost lots of weight that way. It's really confusing.
Rachael, 34

I want to go on a diet, and my doctor has told me it will ease my symptoms, but there are so many out there and they all sound so convincing. I wish someone would just tell me which diet is right for me.
Marion, 30

It's uncertain whether there is one definitive PCOS diet. 'One woman with PCOS may find that a low carbohydrate diet helps her, but another may not. We are all individuals and the important thing is to find a diet that is acceptable and sustainable for you.
PCOS expert Dr Adam Balen, consultant Obstetrician and Gynaecologist and Specialist in Reproductive Medicine and Surgery at Leeds General Infirmary, UK

The Diet Plan Guide

Following a diet plan can seem like a good idea when you're leading a busy life and want to change your eating habits – but which popular diet plans are actually PCOS-fighting, and which are fad crash diets that won't help your PCOS in the long term? For a discussion of low-carb and high protein diets, turn to page 190; the table below is a basic guide to other diets which could be useful for women with PCOS.

A word of warning: don't ever be taken in by diets that claim to help you lose huge amounts of weight in short amounts of time, or diets based on one ingredient ('monodiets') such as cabbage soup or grapefruit – these are not offering a nutritionally-balanced option for long-term health for women with PCOS.

What's the Diet?	Meal replacements
What's the Idea?	Replacing meals with nutritionally-balanced drinks or shakes
Will It Help My PCOS?	May be a healthy short-term solution under the supervision of a nutritionist or doctor. If you choose to try this, be sure to snack on fruits and vegetables to increase your phytochemical intake. Once you've lost the weight, try to go back to eating, not drinking, your food.
What's the Diet?	The Chocolate Diet
What's the Idea?	Created by Sally Ann Voak, chocoholics are divided into six types and each is allocated a diet to cope with their particular issues. The aim is to improve your relationship with chocolate so that you feel more in control.
Will It Help My PCOS?	Certainly could do – if you are addicted to chocolate or other sweet foods, this healthy diet plan can encourage you to deal with your emotional relationship to food.
What's the Diet?	The Omega Diet
What's the Idea?	An eating system based on 12 food units (protein, seeds, nuts, etc.) a day to provide all the nutrients and calories needed, without having to count calories, read labels or weigh and measure amounts. Creator Judith Wells says, 'up to 75 per cent of us are eating too few essential fatty acids, or the wrong balance of them.'

Will It Help My PCOS?	Could be really useful. Women with PCOS do need to ensure that they get enough EFAs; following this eating plan is a good, healthy way of doing this.
What's the Diet?	The Schwarbein principle
What's the Idea?	That food should be thought of in terms of the effect it can have on your hormones, including insulin.
Will It Help My PCOS?	Possibly. The diet recommends avoiding processed carbohydrates in favour of those you can 'pick, gather or milk'. Also emphasizes the importance of 'good' fats: eggs, butter, flaxseed oil, olive oil. The principle is helpful for PCOS symptoms but the diet itself, which emphasizes high-cholesterol foods, would have to be altered to meet the needs of women with PCOS.
What's the Diet?	Detox/fasting
What's the Idea?	Cutting out foods/using detox supplements to help you lose weight/allow your body to use its own energy reserves.
Will It Help My PCOS?	Fasting stresses the body, even in the short term. It slows the metabolism and may throw blood-sugar levels into chaos. Do not try this unless under the supervision of your healthcare practitioner.
What's the Diet?	The Zone diet
What's the Idea?	Based on a ratio of at least 1:1, though can go up to 2:1, carbs to protein at every meal, advocating

	healthy, fresh foods rich in Omega-3s and vegetarian protein.
Will It Help My PCOS?	Can be very helpful in controlling insulin resistance and maintaining a healthy weight, promoting a good balance of carbs and proteins and providing essential vitamins and minerals.

Fad diets look simple, and sometimes they can give short-term results. But no matter how sophisticated a fad diet sounds, the great majority operate on one doomed, ill-fated tactic: drastic calorie reduction. These doomed diets usually deprive your body of essential nutrients, exacerbate your symptoms, may trigger overeating due to deprivation and often make it more difficult to lose weight in the long run. They may even add complications you don't need and put your health at risk.

Once you are on your healthy eating path and reaping the benefits, it's time to think about stage 2: your diet and lifestyle detox.

The PCOS Detox Boost

There are many things in our day-to-day lives which can make the symptoms of PCOS worse, or push a woman who has PCO (without any symptoms) into developing PCOS (with symptoms).

Every day, a sea of potentially hormone-disturbing toxins surrounds you, from environmental chemicals in solvents, plastics and adhesives to toxins in makeup, moisturizers, nail polish, hair dyes and shampoos. Even food and soil are inundated with pesticides and herbicides, not forgetting the contaminants and parasites in the water you drink, and the chemicals and additives added to refined processed food which detract from the nutritional content of the food.

Our bodies don't need or want any of these chemicals, and have to work hard to process (metabolize) them and get rid of them (detoxify). In the process of metabolizing these toxins, our bodies lose vital nutrients – nutrients we need to feel healthy and beat the symptoms of PCOS.

WHERE DO THESE TOXINS COME FROM?

Literally anywhere, from pesticide residues on food to the environmental poisons in our air and water, and the high-sugar, preserved and processed fast foods in our diet. The landmark 1989 Kellogg Report stated that there are now over 1,000 newly-synthesized compounds introduced each year, which amounts to around 20 new chemicals a week. But many of these chemicals are not ordinary chemicals. They are petrochemicals, found in pesticides, plastics, household cleaners, car exhausts and even makeup. Petrochemicals are known as xenobiotics or xenoestrogens.

Hormone-disturbing Chemicals

Environmental scientist Theo Colburn first brought xenoestrogens to the public's attention. Xenoestrogens, or endocrine-disrupting chemicals (EDC), are widely recognized as highly toxic in the smallest doses. Most importantly for women with PCOS, they are characterized as 'hormone-disrupters' because these petrochemicals have a molecular structure similar to the hormone oestrogen.

EDCs interfere with the natural process of your hormones, preventing them from producing the natural response in much the same way that a vehicle parked across an entrance prevents other vehicles from getting out or in. They create hormonal havoc by tricking your body into a condition known as *oestrogen excess* or *oestrogen dominance*. For women with PCOS who are often exposed to chronic levels of oestrogen without the balancing effects of progesterone anyway, oestrogen dominance can trigger a wide variety of PCOS symptoms, from irregular periods to acne, dry hair and weight gain.

In 1999, the Federal Environmental Agency in Germany published a list of pesticides to be confirmed as potential endocrine-disrupters, including pesticides used on food, wood preservatives, paints and plastics. The research necessary to confirm conclusively which chemicals are EDCs is still being carried out, however the Environmental Agency has stated that there should be action to reduce further environmental exposure while this research is on going.

There is little scientific evidence about how a poor diet and exposure to EDCs affect women with PCOS, but we know enough to suggest that exposure to potentially hormone-disrupting toxins and eating an unhealthy diet don't benefit those who are well and healthy, let alone someone who may have a condition or potential hormonal imbalance like PCOS. 'Humans are exposed daily to chemicals that have been shown or suggested to have hormone-disrupting properties,' states a June 2000 Royal Society Report. 'Despite the uncertainty, it is prudent to minimize the exposure to humans, especially pregnant women, to endocrine-disrupting chemicals.' Taking measures to avoid hormone-disrupting chemicals in the food we eat and in our environment can help reduce the toxic load for women with PCOS, and protect us from added hormonal disturbance.

Research in 2002 from Brunel University reported on a five-year study which found that sex changes in male fish in some UK rivers were caused by synthetic oestrogens in the river water (which contained sewage waste which included the urine of women on the Pill). Dr Susan Toblin was quoted as saying, 'One could argue we are living in a sea of oestrogen, a chemical cocktail, and therefore I think there are real reasons to be worried about health and fertility.'

YOUR BODY'S IN-HOUSE DETOX SYSTEM

Your liver, kidneys and adrenal glands work extremely hard to keep your hormones functioning efficiently and you feeling healthy. They are crucial for the removal of potentially harmful toxins which can disrupt your hormonal systems and trigger the symptoms of PCOS.

Your *liver* is a chemical clearing workaholic. It cleans one-and-a-half quarts of blood every minute of the day, so that other organs can be nourished by purified blood. It also neutralizes toxic wastes, sending them off to the next detox organ, the kidneys, for elimination. The liver also removes excess hormones (such as oestrogen), thereby maintaining hormonal balance, produces enzymes and amino acids to metabolize fat, proteins and carbs, stores nutrients, makes and processes cholesterol, produces bile during the digestive process for fat metabolism, and regulates blood-sugar levels for energy.

Alcohol, drugs, fatty foods, highly refined foods, smoking, drugs, the Pill
and other environmental toxins, from pesticides and exhaust fumes to
hair sprays and petrol, can overload the liver. Whether you have PCOS or
not, if toxins clog up the liver's detoxification pathways, blood-sugar
levels start to fluctuate, toxins start to find their way into your circulatory
system and excess hormones can't be cleared from your system,
resulting in hair loss and irregular periods.

The skin, like the liver, is a major detoxifying organ, so waste materials
exit through the skin's pores and show up on your face, hair and nails,
causing wrinkles, acne, blotchy skin, blemishes, bad hair days, split nails
and white blotches on your nails – all clear warning signs that vital
nutrients are lacking.

Your *kidneys* and bladder work harmoniously with your liver to eliminate
waste from your system. The kidneys help your system keep the right
amount of minerals, while pulling out unwanted elements like nitrogen,
salts and certain chemicals. When the filtering is complete, urine flows
from the kidneys to the bladder where it is eliminated.

When your liver can't cope with too many toxins, the excess passes into
your bloodstream and to your kidneys. But your kidneys are not designed
to detoxify waste, as your liver does. Consequently the toxic substances
move to the urinary tract where they can cause yeast infections. Your
skin is also forced to do double time in the elimination process, which
can cause rashes, acne and other skin conditions.

Situated on top of your kidneys, your *adrenal glands* are on the alert every
second of the day, responding to the pressures affecting you. In order to
cope, the adrenals manufacture hormones such as adrenaline and
cortisol, which keep blood sugar in check so that you receive the energy
you need. The more your adrenals are under siege because of physical,
emotional or environmental stress, the greater likelihood of burn-out or
adrenal exhaustion. When this occurs, too much cortisol is produced,
which in turn can trigger testosterone production and the familiar
symptoms of PCOS.

Your *lymph system* is also crucial to your body's detox processes. Lymph, a liquid produced by the lymph glands in various parts of your body, absorbs dead cells, excess fluids and other waste products from foods and takes them to the lymph nodes. Here the waste is filtered and eventually fed into the blood and on to one of the eliminatory organs – skin, liver or kidneys – to be passed out via perspiration, faeces or urine.

Poor lymph drainage due to excess waste results in a build-up of fluids containing waste products. This waste can become toxic and stagnant, and eventually will make you feel bloated and tired. In addition, tissues can be damaged due to excess fluid.

What Can You Do?

There are two things you can do to help keep your liver, kidneys and adrenals in good working order and protect yourself from toxins:

1 Give them nutritional support from a healthy diet. Nutrients can help process, transform or eliminate toxins and excess hormones through the liver's detoxification pathways. A healthy diet can help you prevent, control and repair the damage toxins have caused, while working to restore hormonal balance in your body.
2 Reduce the amount of toxins in your food, chemical home cleaners, cosmetics, plastic and water supply, in order to allow your body's natural detoxification systems to function optimally and regulate your hormones.

DETOXIFICATION

There are many detox programmes recommending you drink only water and vegetable juice for a number of days to cleanse your system, and then add in other foods over a week or so. These aren't usually a good idea, because they slow metabolism and are very hard to stick to.

You don't really need to go on fasts, retreats or harsh regimes or take supplements to protect yourself from toxins. The best way to protect against toxicity is to keep your body's own self-purifying system in good working order, by eating well, reducing the number of toxins you put into your body, and following these recommendations:

1 Drink pure water.
2 Eat healthy, fresh food.
3 Always read the labels.
4 Go organic.
5 Cut down on caffeine and alcohol.
6 Stop smoking.
7 Ditch the 'bad' fats.
8 Try chemical-free living.
9 Reduce your stress.
10 Get enough sleep.

Now let's take a closer look at each of these.

1) Water, Water

Without water, you can't survive. Making sure that the water you drink is pure and clean is a good first step. The World Health Organization has claimed that 80 per cent of world's illnesses would be eliminated if we all drank pure water. Water replenishes, cleanses, rejuvenates and restores your liver, kidneys and adrenals. It is the most important item in any detox plan. We've also seen in the previous chapter how important it is for women with PCOS to ensure an adequate intake of fluid.

But where do we find pure water?

The standard purification techniques used by most water companies remove the bugs from the water but do not remove all the dissolved chemicals. It is estimated that as many as 60,000 different chemicals now contaminate our water supplies. In attempts to clean the water, other chemicals are sometimes added, including chlorine and aluminium.

Not only may these chemicals be toxic in their own right, but chlorine may react with organic waste to form compounds which can increase the risk of cancer of the colon, rectum and bladder.

The recognition that much of our tap water is contaminated has seen the boom in bottled-water sales. According to Professor Larry Laudan in his book *Danger Ahead*, however, there's a one-in-four chance that the next batch of bottled water you drink will be nothing more than tap water which has been passed through a filter.

There is also little need to drink mineral water to obtain the minerals we need for our bodies. While this type of water does contain essential trace minerals, it also contains calcium carbonate, which our bodies need but cannot absorb in a desirable way from water. This calcium carbonate can contribute to blocking of the arteries and to arthritis, rheumatism, gout and indigestion. The best source of minerals is vegetables grown in mineral-rich soil.

Distilled water isn't much better. The process of distillation can concentrate some compounds and remove essential trace elements. For water to be pure, it must be double distilled. Few companies do this.

What to Do?

Ideally, all drinking water should be purified in the home. You can do this with water filters and water filter systems. The quickest and easiest are water-filter jugs, readily available from department stores and health food shops. Use the filtered water for cooking as well as for hot and cold drinks. Bear in mind that filters can become breeding grounds for bacteria, so regularly replacing the filter and cleaning the filter-housing is essential. A good quality filter should eliminate, or greatly reduce, the levels of heavy metals such as lead, cadmium and mercury, fluoride and chlorine, and remove any adverse tastes, colours and odours in the water.

If you want to go to the next level of convenience you can buy plumbed-in carbon filters to use at your kitchen sink. These are effective at removing chlorine, heavy metals and many organic compounds. However they may not be so successful at removing nitrates and bacterial contaminants.

A more sophisticated type of filter called a *reverse osmosis system* can be fitted to your mains water system at home. It forces water under pressure through a semi-permeable membrane and allows you to use as much water as you want. It is fairly effective and inexpensive to run, but the storage tank takes up a lot of space and needs regular maintenance. Any system you buy should be able to reduce the contamination to less than 10 parts per million. That's about as clean as you can get. If installing a system like this is too expensive, or you live in rented accommodation, portable filters which use cartridges to help get rid of chemicals are your best option.

Alternatively, buy water bottled in glass rather than plastic. Plastic bottled water can increase the amount of toxins because plastic compounds are leached from the bottle into the water. Or drink cooled boiled tap water – this at least gets rid of the bacteria and removes the amount of limescale you are drinking in.

Hot and Cold

If you are still using tap water, and suspect that you have lead pipes, use only the cold for drinking and cooking. There is a greater probability that the hot water contains chemicals, like lead and asbestos. Let the cold water tap run for a few minutes until it is as cold as it can get to flush out the pipes. The longer it sits in the pipes, the higher the level of pollutants.

2) Eat Healthy, Fresh Food

Eating fresh foods not only helps to reduce the amount of pollutants in your body, it boosts the nutritional support to your in-house detox system. It also reduces the amount of refined foodstuffs you take in – sometimes these can be so refined that they can actually become toxic. Your body sees ingredients like pure sugar, salt and hydrogenated or chemically processed fats, or food colourings, preservatives and additives, as unwanted toxins.

Taste and visual inspection aren't enough these days to separate healthy from unhealthy foods. Some of the most dangerous pollutants are invisible and without taste. You need to know as much as possible about *where* your food and drink come from and *how* they have been treated.

Processed, ready-cooked, canned and refined foods often contain high levels of hidden salt, sugar, artificial sweeteners and saturated fat, as well as hydrogenated fats which prevent the body absorbing the essential fatty acids crucial for brain, hormone, skin and emotional health. Sugars will be stored as central body fat and laid down within the blood vessels, producing a furring of the arteries or atherosclerosis. Additional salt will tend to increase blood pressure. We've seen already that high blood pressure and increasing body fat, especially around the waist, are things to be avoided because they carry with them severe health risks, especially for women with PCOS.

You can cut down on or eliminate sugar easily by avoiding many sweet foods. Good foods to replace sugar treats include fruit slices, pretzels (unsalted!), popcorn, rice cakes and mixed nuts, vegetable sticks, salads, almonds, granola, yogurt, wine gums and dark chocolate with a high cocoa content. A diet high in whole grains and other complex carbohydrates, vegetables and protein foods can also help curb your cravings for sugary foods.

Healthy Eating Ideas

You may feel that you haven't got the time to prepare fresh foods all the time, but there are easy ways you can incorporate more and more of them into your diet:

- The useful life of fresh foods can be extended by storing them in the fridge or freezer.
- You could prepare your meals at the weekend and then store them in your freezer to be eaten during the week.
- You could order fresh food every few days via a mail-order, internet or phone service.

– Soups made from fresh vegetables, with grains and legumes, are easy to make and keep.

– A casserole is a great way to include vegetables, grains and meat in your diet.

– Salads are quick and easy to prepare, so keep the salad crisper in your fridge well-stocked – or you can buy ready-made salad packets if you are in a rush.

– Tiered steamers can be used to cook fish and vegetables at the same time.

– You can add your own fresh vegetables and toppings to pizza bases.

– Wholemeal bread with low-fat fillings like chicken or tuna along with a side salad makes for a quick and easy light meal.

– Keep fresh fruit handy, even at work.

Healthy Cooking Tips

– Fried and even heavily charcoal-grilled foods can produce antibodies and free radicals which can damage cell membranes. These cooking methods should be avoided. When frying, add a small amount of water to cold-pressed oil and never let the oil get so hot that it smokes. Try grilling or baking instead of frying.

– To avoid nutrient loss, lightly steam vegetables in a little water.

– With organic foods you need only scrub the skins, as many of the nutrients are concentrated under the skin. With non-organic vegetables, try vegetable-washing products (available from health stores) or soak them in a bowl of water with a capful of cider vinegar to wash out impurities. If this isn't possible, peel fruits and vegetables before using them. Remove and discard the outer leaves of cabbage, lettuce and other greens.

– Avoid all aluminium cookware, as this is a heavy toxic metal which can enter food through the cooking process. The same applies to wrapping foods in aluminium foil. The best cookware to use is cast iron, enamel, glass or stainless steel.

– As far as possible, avoid foods and drinks in plastic containers or wrapped in plastic. Don't store any fatty foods (such as cheeses or meats) in plastic wrap. Remove food from plastic packaging as soon as possible – especially before microwaving.

Detox Superfoods

Certain foods and drinks are thought to strengthen and improve liver action, cleanse blood, support the kidneys, improve digestion and so aid detoxification.

For the liver: apples, artichokes, asparagus, beetroot, berries, blue-green algae, broccoli, brown rice, buckwheat, cabbage, carrots, celery, chicory, dandelion, fennel, garlic, kelp, leeks, lemons, lemon juice or cider vinegar in a cup of hot water (adding honey makes the drink even more cleansing for the bowels), millet, oat bran, oily fish, onions, parsley, parsnips, sesame oil and seeds, spinach, strawberries, sunflower seeds, turmeric, watercress, wholefoods (such as quinoa and amaranth). Chlorophyll-rich spices such as dill, mint, tarragon and thyme are time-honoured detoxifiers that nourish the bloodstream while assisting the body in the digestive process.

For the kidneys: asparagus, beetroot, blackberries, broccoli, cabbage, celery, cranberries, eggs, fennel, garlic, grains (buckwheat, barley, millet), grapes, green beans, horseradish, kidney beans, leeks, lettuce, lovage, marrows, melons, nettles, oranges, oysters, papaya, parsley, peas, pineapple juice, pulses, radishes, raspberries, rice, sea vegetables, sesame seeds, swedes, tarragon, tamari sauce, turnips, vervain, walnuts, watercress

For the adrenal glands: the kidneys and adrenals are connected, so all foods, herbs and spices that can strengthen the kidneys will also strengthen the adrenals. In addition it is important for the adrenals that you consume foods high in potassium such as bananas, raisins, peanuts, garlic, chicken and carrots, and avoid foods high in sodium. Foods rich in vitamin C, such as apples, oranges and green vegetables, are also recommended as this vitamin is necessary for the production of adrenal hormones.

Herbs and Supplements for Your Liver and Kidneys

A multivitamin and mineral complex with vitamin B complex and selenium and zinc is recommended, as well as vitamin C and vitamin E supplements. Other nutritional supplements to support the liver include: glutathione, glutamine, lecithin, cysteine, and taurine.

Alfalfa, burdock, chamomile, dandelion, lemon, red clover, rose-hip teas and green tea can also rejuvenate the liver and help you gently detox. Sip some throughout the day.

Milk thistle is another excellent herb for the liver. A number of studies have shown that it can increase the number of new liver cells to replace old damaged ones.[1]

Caster oil, applied externally, can be used to stimulate the liver and draw out toxins from the body. Apply slightly warmed oil to your stomach with a flannel and leave for one hour.

To keep your kidneys in good working order, certain herbal teas are of great benefit. The leaves and flowers of goldenrod can be made into a tea that is drunk up to three times a day (it is available in ready-made preparations). Other beneficial herbs and spices include cinnamon, cloves, buchu tea, nettle tea and parsley.

Numerous herbs support adrenal function, but the most notable are the ginsengs, which a qualified practitioner should prescribe.

(For a liver-boosting salad recipe, see page 110.)

You can undertake a naturopathic detox using psyllium seeds and bentonite clay. Some naturopaths mix the clay and seeds together in one drink. Psyllium seeds are a soluble form of fibre. By taking 3 to 4 grams of psyllium a day you can lower cholesterol levels by 20 per cent in a matter of weeks. Psyllium can also help metabolize fat more efficiently.

Psyllium can reduce food cravings – by mixing 3 to 4 grams in a glass of juice and drinking it before meals you can feel quite full even before eating. However, do *not* use this powerful combination without supervision by a naturopath.

Eastern Detox Systems

Ayurvedic Medicine
Ayurveda is an ancient medical system still practised today throughout India, Sri Lanka and Nepal. The system is derived from the ancient wisdom of the Vedas and is based on harmonizing the three *Doshas* or energy types – Vata, Pitta and Kapha – which balance our diet, lifestyle and general health. Vata is thought to control movement, Pitta is responsible for metabolism and digestion, and Kapha governs the structure of the body. Through balancing the Doshas you can cultivate *Ojas* – well-being, health and vitality in both mind and body.

Let's look at some Ayurvedic energy-balancing techniques for strengthening digestion:

- Eat in a settled and quiet atmosphere.
- Take a few minutes to rest quietly after a meal.
- Always sit down to eat.
- Don't eat when you are upset.
- Avoid foods and drinks that are too hot or too cold.
- Don't talk while chewing your food.
- Take your time over a meal.
- Leave three to six hours between each meal (this does not include light snacks, which can be taken more often).
- Eat as much fresh food as possible.

Techniques to eliminate toxins and purify the body include:

❋ **Devote one day a week to an entirely liquid diet to strengthen digestion and eliminate toxins. This isn't fasting, as anything can be included in your diet as long as it is liquefied. To liquefy a food,** simply place it in a blender and add warm water. You may take the liquids or liquefied foods as often as you like during the day. Soups, herbal teas, fresh fruits and vegetables and grains which have been blended with water are best suited to this routine.

❋ Sip hot water frequently throughout the day. For best results the water should be sipped every 30 minutes.

The herbal supplements recommended by Ayurvedic doctors are primarily intended to strengthen the mind/body connection and rectify the energy imbalances that create disease. An Ayurvedic herb prescription might include the following to benefit digestion:

Amalaki	Relieves irritation throughout the gastrointestinal system and, important for women with PCOS, stabilizes blood-sugar irregularities
Bibihitaki	Has a strong but safe laxative effect
Chitrak	Reduces the accumulation of toxins by preventing stagnation in the gastrointestinal system
Lavanga or cloves	Have energizing effects which can stimulate digestion

Chinese Medicine

Traditional Chinese medicine taps into nature's wonderful system of balance by using food, healing teas, herbs and spices to balance your body's energy, cooling it down in spring and summer and firing it up in the autumn and winter.

The following herbs are commonly used by Chinese medical herbalists to detox the liver, kidneys and adrenals: calendula, chamomile, dandelion root, echinacea, lemon balm, liquorice root, stinging nettles, garlic, cayenne, sarsaparilla, ginger, red clover, sage and thyme.

A Chinese doctor would regard PCOS as a sign that your whole body is in a state of imbalance, and it is this imbalance rather than the symptoms that would be treated. The theory is that any kind of hormonal balance indicates a blockage of energy flow which needs to be unblocked through diet and lifestyle changes, herbal remedies and perhaps acupuncture.

According to Ruth Delman, founder of the Chi Health Centre in London, 'a healthy diet is the starting point for treating women with PCOS.' At the Chi Centre, patients with PCOS are advised to stay away from sugary foods and dairy products and to avoid hot and spicy foods, chocolate, caffeine and wheat which overwork the digestive system and create hormonal imbalance. Dietary recommendations include lots of fruit and vegetables and an adequate intake of fish and protein. Priti Patel, practitioner at the Chi Centre, says that PCOS is linked to a kidney dysfunction and hormone imbalance, and that treatment would involve toning the kidneys and restoring hormonal balance: 'Yiyi ren for water retention, Hawthorn fruit for the digestive system, Angelica root, Dang gui and Dan shen to improve circulation are the most common herbal remedies,' she says, 'but the prescription and dose would vary from woman to woman.'

Warning: Herbs can be powerful healers and detoxifiers, but it is important that you seek information and qualified assistance before using them. Always seek the advice of your doctor or a trained nutritionist or herbalist before taking any herbs or supplements. Do not take herbs or supplements if you are pregnant or breastfeeding. (For more advice and information about herbs and supplements, see Chapter 8.)

3) Read the Labels

We should all be worried about additives in our foods because they have been linked to a variety of health problems including headaches, asthma, allergies and hyperactivity in kids. But for women with PCOS these additives – in the form of colourings, preservatives, flavour-enhancers, emulsifiers, stabilizers and thickeners – can add to the toxic load and increase the likelihood of irregular periods, acne, hair loss, weight gain and fatigue, by blocking the body's own detox system.

We are fortunate today that food manufacturers are required to list the ingredients in their products. And recently in the UK, the Government's Food Standards Agency enforced new rules to stop manufacturers of processed food confusing us with inaccurate descriptions and labelling lies. Start reading labels and getting used to spotting hidden ingredients in your food. Also watch out for alternative names. For instance, sodium is just another name for salt, animal fat is saturated fat and transfatty acid is another name for hydrogenated fat. As for sugar, the pseudonyms this one goes by are legion, and include: sucrose, fructose, dextrose, corn syrup, malt syrup and maple syrup. Artificial sweeteners such as mannitol, sorbitol, xylitol, acesulfame K, saccharin and aspartame have no calories and are used mainly in diet drinks and desserts and table-top sweeteners. They should all be avoided.

Colourings

A dangerous class of additives, and one of the easiest to avoid, are the dyes capable of interacting with and damaging your immune system, speeding up ageing, exacerbating symptoms of PCOS and even pushing you in the direction of cancer. Steer clear of foods made with artificial colours. Watch out for labels with any of the following terms: 'artificial colour added' 'FD and C red no 3' (or the words 'green', 'blue' or 'yellow' followed by any number), or simply 'colour added' with no explanation.

Many synthetic food dyes which had been deemed safe have turned out to be carcinogenic. Some dyes approved in Europe are not considered safe in the US, and vice versa. You don't add dyes to the food you cook at home, so why eat them in the foods that you buy?

Names to Look Out for
Tartrazine (E102)
Quinoline yellow (E104)
Sunset yellow (E110)
Beetroot red (E162)
Caramel (E150)

Some foods contain natural colours obtained from plants. These are safe. The most common is *annatto*, from the reddish seed of a tropical tree. Annatto is often added to cheese to make it orange, or to butter to make it yellow. A red pigment obtained from beets, a green one from chlorella, and carotene from carrots are also safe.

Preservatives

The main function of preservatives is to extend a food's shelf-life. Citric acid and ascorbic acid (vitamin C) are natural antioxidants added to a number of foods, and they are safe, but synthetic additives such as BHA and BHT may not be. They may promote the carcinogenic changes in cells caused by other substances. Alum, an aluminium compound, is used in brands of many pickles to increase crispness and is also found in some antacids and baking powder. Aluminium has no place in human nutrition and you should avoid ingesting it.

Nitrites
Nitrites are a type of preservative added to many cured meats. They can create highly carcinogenic substances called nitrosamines in the body. It is best to avoid hot dogs, sausages, lunch meats and other products containing sodium nitrate or other nitrites – these foods are also high in saturated fat, dense animal protein and salt.

Monosodium glutamate (MSG) a natural product long used in East Asian cooking is added to many manufactured foods as a flavour-enhancer. It is an unnecessary source of additional sodium in the diet and can cause allergic reactions. Omit MSG from recipes, don't buy products containing it, and when eating out in Chinese restaurants request that food be made without it.

Nitrites and Nitrates (E249-52)	Found in processed meats, such as sausages, bacon and ham, and in smoked fish
Benzoic acid and benzoates (E210-19)	Found in soft drinks, beer, salad creams
Sulphur dioxide and sulphites (E220-29)	Found in dried fruits, fruit-based pie fillings, relishes
Ascorbic acid/ascorbates (E300-4)	Found in fruit juices, fruit jams, tinned fruit
BHA/BHT (E320-21)	Found in foods where rancidity needs to be prevented, e.g. crisps, biscuits and fruit pies

Flavour-enhancers
Monosodium glutamate or MSG (621)
Monopotassium glutamate (622)
Sodium inosinate (631)

Emulsifiers, Stabilizers and Thickeners

These are found in sauces, soups, breads, biscuits, cakes, frozen desserts, ice cream, margarine and other spreads, jams, chocolate and milk shakes.

Guar gum (E412)
Gum arabic (E414)
Pectins (E440)
Cellulose (E460)
Lecithin (E322)
Glycerol (E422)

It can be difficult to understand labels that list a lot of long chemical names. A good general rule is simply to avoid products whose chemical ingredients outnumber the familiar ones. Some chemicals are quite harmless, for instance ammonium bicarbonate, malic acid, fumaric acid, lactic acid, lecithin, xanthan, guar gums, calcium chloride, monocalcium phosphate and monopotassium phosphate. More and more manufacturers are clearing up their products as people get more concerned about toxins in their food and you will increasingly see 'no artificial sweeteners' or 'no artificial ingredients'. This is helpful. If you can't understand a label, though, or there's barely enough room for all the chemical ingredients, leave the product on the shelf.

Many processed foods also come in packets ready to warm up before heating. They are stored wrapped in plastic and aluminium. Both of these storage methods will add additional non-food chemicals into your food, especially when heated. Cans of fizzy drink contain six times the amount of aluminium compared to the same beverages in glass bottles. There is always a small amount of residue that dissolves into drinks from the lining of a can or from a plastic bottle. Glass bottles are much better than plastic. Also avoid heating food wrapped in plastic.

4) Organic Is Better

If you have PCOS and want to reduce the chemical load on your body, organic food is really a good way to help yourself. The production of organic food is governed by strict standards. In organic farming the use of chemical fertilizers and pesticides is avoided (a good thing, because many of these are hormone-disrupters), and animals and poultry are raised in natural conditions on organically-farmed land and must not be treated with antibiotics on a routine basis.

This means that not only does your food contain fewer chemical residues than non-organic food, it also reduces the amount of chemicals being washed through the soil into the water supply. It makes sense not just for PCOS symptoms but, according to research from the UK Soil Association, for your overall health now and in the long term.

Most supermarkets sell organic produce, though it can be expensive. Try and buy just one item a week to get into the habit of looking at organic food as an investment for your health. You could also get boxes of seasonal fruit and vegetables delivered to your door; there are mail order services which can provide everything organic, from milk to mushrooms.

In the US there are many organic farmers' markets which sell directly to the public, cutting out the middle man and cutting the price. These are starting to catch on in the UK. Contact local government offices or your neighbourhood health food store about getting local, cheaper organic foods (see Chapter 12).

Make sure the food you buy is really organic by looking for certification labels from well-respected organizations such as the Soil Association in the UK or Earth Source Greens in the US.

If you can't find or afford much organic food, remember that eating lots of fruits and vegetables, whether organic or not, is a great step towards boosting your health. If you can get organic food even just occasionally it can help to enhance your health even more.

5) Cut Down on Caffeine and Alcohol

Coffee beans, tea leaves and cocoa beans all contain caffeine. Although you may think of this as a harmless part of your diet, caffeine can have a significant effect on your body. Like sugar, caffeine overstimulates the adrenals; persistent and chronic caffeine consumption weakens them. A cycle develops where greater and greater amounts are needed to achieve the familiar high, and symptoms such as headaches and indigestion can occur if we don't get our fix.

Caffeine is a potent drug used in pain-relieving medications such as headache and cold remedies. Caffeine-containing drinks are popular because of the lift they give us, helping us to wake in the morning or muster that extra bit of energy to face an hour of work late at night. Many women also find that caffeine helps to suppress their appetite, making dieting easier. However, caffeine can also disturb your sleep pattern and cause withdrawal symptoms if you vary your intake from day to day. And if you have PCOS, caffeine can trigger problems with blood sugar.

Tea and coffee also deplete your body of essential nutrients. Tea, for example, contains tannin which can stop you absorbing vital nutrients, like iron. This means that if you drink tea at mealtimes you could eat a nutritious meal and waste these vital nutrients by excreting them unabsorbed. Caffeine has also been linked to infertility. Several research studies have suggested that drinking as little as two to four cups of tea or coffee a day may delay conception.[2] Finally, there are the toxic chemicals used in growing and processing coffee.

So does all this mean you have to give up caffeine altogether if you have PCOS?

In general, the weight of scientific opinion seems to support the idea that a moderate amount of tea and coffee does not significantly compromise your health or fertility and, according to a study published by the US National Institutes of Health and the American Heart Association, drinking tea may even reduce the risk of heart disease by improving the functioning of artery walls.

So overall, it seems that you don't need to cut out tea, chocolate and coffee altogether, you just need to cut your intake of caffeine and caffeinated drinks to one or two cups a day, or to switch to herbal or fruit teas.

Tea Is Good for Your Heart

According to a recent study, Dutch scientists suggest that drinking two cups of tea a day cuts the risk of developing heart disease by over 50 per cent.

Tea, like chocolate and apples, contains chemicals called *catechins* which are thought to reduce the level of harmful substances in the arteries and protect against heart disease. Tea can be drunk black or with milk, as the milk proteins do not block the uptake of catechins into the body.

Healthy Alternatives

If you have PCOS, why not try fruit or herbal teas instead of tea and coffee? As well as being caffeine-free, these teas can aid relaxation. Decaffeinated alternatives are not really a wise option, as we have no idea which chemicals are involved in the decaffeination process (although there is a revolutionary new water-decaffeination process used by some organic companies). If you want to try decaffeinated products, your best option is to go for organic decaffeinated teas and coffees which don't have chemicals in them.

There are a number of herbal teas which can be both stimulating and refreshing. The roasted herbal roots, including: barley, chicory and dandelion, are most popular. Grain coffee such as Rombouts, Postum, Pero and Wilson's Heritage are also favoured among coffee-drinkers, while ginseng root teas is recommended by some. Herbal teas made from lemon grass, peppermint, gingerroot, red clover and comfrey, rosehip, apple, hibiscus, clover flower and nettles can be comforting and nourishing without the depleting side-effects of caffeine. Chamomile tea is good for inducing calm and sleep; peppermint is good for indigestion.

It is best to withdraw gradually from caffeine to avoid headaches. Lower your caffeine intake by drinking grain coffee-blends, or diluted or smaller amounts of regular coffee. Another approach is to first substitute black tea, which has less caffeine than coffee and can be tapered off more easily. If headaches occur, increase your water intake and keep eating a healthy balanced diet. This should ease the withdrawal symptoms.

Alcohol

Alcohol can interfere with hormonal health. Too much isn't a good idea if you have PCOS, for several reasons:

– Alcohol exerts an oestrogen-like action and can be thought of as adding to the body's oestrogen load.

– Research has shown that women who drink heavily stop ovulating and menstruating and take longer to conceive.[3]

– Alcohol is a source of empty calories and, since alcohol often replaces nutrition, the body receives fewer essential nutrients. For instance, alcohol can stop you absorbing zinc, which is crucial for hormonal health.

– Alcoholic drinks contain a lot of sugar and are a source of refined carbohydrates.

– Alcohol molecules are so small and easy to absorb that they get assimilated before other foods, directly entering the bloodstream for a quick effect. Beer, wine and mixed drinks can cause rapid fluctuations of the blood sugar. Carbohydrate metabolism is affected by alcohol; this can lead to hypoglycemia and diabetes.

– The liver is the only organ that metabolizes alcohol, either converting it into energy or storing it as fat. When there is excess consumption this can interfere with the liver's normal functioning and make it less able to get rid of excess circulating hormones. The liver is also the organ that clears out any excess hormones. If you drink too much alcohol, this can lead to hormonal imbalance.

– Fat builds up in the liver. Since alcohol converts to fat, obesity also often occurs with high alcohol use.

The risks of alcohol are directly related to the amount you drink, and the time period over which you drink. High-risk use would be having more than five drinks daily, moderate-risk use three to four drinks a day, and low-risk one or two drinks daily. But women with diabetes, hypertension or heart disease should avoid alcohol altogether. If you have PCOS, you should also avoid it or cut it down to fewer than five drinks a week. A study of 430 women demonstrated that drinking more than five drinks a week could stop women conceiving.[4] The fact is that alcohol can interfere with hormonal health, and the more you drink the worse the impact is.

We would suggest that while you are trying to bring your symptoms under control, avoiding alcohol is very helpful. When cutting down, follow the healthy diet guidelines in Chapter 2, have some nourishment every two to three hours and drink lots of water to help clear your liver and cleanse your body of toxins. Once you feel fitter and healthier there is no reason why you shouldn't enjoy drinking alcohol in moderation again (say one glass of wine, spirits or beer a day). There are also many lower-alcohol wines and spirits available today, and an increasing number of organic options available in supermarkets and through mail-order companies.

Red Wine, Beer and Spirits

A small amount of alcohol may have some beneficial effects for women with PCOS. It is thought that one or two units of red wine a day can decrease the risk of heart disease. Like exercise, red wine increases the levels of good (HDL) cholesterol in the blood. It contains bioflavonoids, which together with the alcohol is cardio-protective. If you have a low level of HDL (good cholesterol), one or two glasses of red wine a day can help raise it. But do remember that exercise can achieve the same desired effect, and should be your first port of call as exercise does not have the additional negative effects that alcohol has.

Beer and spirits may have just as many health benefits as wine, according to a study published in the *Journal of Epidemiology and Community Health*. Researchers believe that beer, spirits and wine may have a positive effect on your immune system. Previous studies have shown that beer is rich in vitamin B_6, which prevents the build-up of the harmful chemicals that can cause heart disease. But again, the research is based on moderate to low alcohol intake.

6) Stop Smoking

Cigarette smoking is the biggest cause of preventable disease, yet probably the most difficult addiction to deal with. Passive smoking, too, has its risks. Just 30 minutes in the company of smokers can damage your heart by reducing its ability to pump blood, according to research published in the *Journal of the American Medical Association* (January, 1998).

Smoking is a significant anti-nutrient. It reduces the level of vitamin C in the bloodstream. Smokers also have high levels of cadmium, a heavy toxic metal that can stop the utilization of zinc, needed for a healthy menstrual cycle. Scientists at Boston Massachusetts General Hospital have also found that smoking can trigger infertility. It is also linked to menstrual irregularities, early menopause, heart disease and poor health in general.

I've always had irregular periods because of my PCOS, so I didn't think that the menopause would affect me. This wasn't the case. I got everything – the hot sweats, the loss of interest in sex, vaginal dryness, weight gain and terrible mood changes. I don't have hormonal therapy for my PCOS, so I wasn't going to take drugs for the menopause, either.

So far I've managed to keep the symptoms of both the menopause and PCOS at bay by cleaning up my diet – cutting down on sugar and eliminating caffeine, alcohol and really fatty foods. As soon as I started to include oestrogen-containing foods in my diet, like soya, tofu and almonds, the hot flushes stopped. I've also stopped smoking completely, and exercise every day for at least half an hour. I thought at first I'd never be able to keep to this routine (I've smoked a pack or two of fags a day since I was 19) but I haven't had a cigarette in years. If I don't exercise I feel sluggish and irritable. And I could never go back to smoking. I was always tired, unwell and stressed when I smoked and, apart from the fact that I know smoking can make my symptoms worse, my daughter had her first child, a little girl called Heather, and I want to be around to see her grow up.
Heather, 46

A UK report published in 2000 by Health Secretary Alan Milburn revealed that over 600 chemicals are allowed into cigarettes, some of which may seem quite bizarre, like the radioactive material polonium acetone (used to make paint-stripper), butane (a form of lighter fuel) and ammonia (found in toilet cleaners). So it's not just nicotine and cadmium that add to the detox load. Health risks increase dramatically if you are a smoker and take the Pill, as many women with PCOS do to reduce their symptoms, because both smoking and the oral contraceptive pill leach the body of the essential nutrients you need to beat the symptoms of

PCOS. So if you have PCOS and you are a smoker, you should consider why you are taking something into your body which can make your symptoms worse.

Your liver and lungs can regenerate themselves if you give them time off from alcohol and smoking and support them with the nutrients they need to thrive. If you want to improve your health, nothing is as effective as stopping smoking completely.

The nutritional strategy for smokers is to increase your intake of wholesome foods – fruits, vegetables and whole grains – and to decrease your intake of fats, cured or pickled food, food additives and alcohol. Research at St George's Hospital Medical School, London, published in the medical journal *Thorax* (January, 2000) has also shown that certain foods, such as apples, can boost lung health and healing capacity. Organic, unfiltered raw apple cider vinegar is a natural tonic for overall health, especially respiratory health. Take a teaspoon in a glass of water every day.

In addition, raw seeds, nuts, legumes, sprouts and other proteins should be consumed. Water is essential to balance out the drying effects of smoking. Since smoking generates an acidic condition in the body, a high-fibre diet helps detoxification by maintaining bowel function.

Supplements and Substitutes

Smoking leaches essential nutrients, so a general multivitamin with additional antioxidant nutrients vitamin A, C, E and selenium is an important part of any smoker's health programme. Cadmium will not leave your body when you stop smoking; it needs to be tackled by supplementing your diet with antioxidant supplements.

Giving Up

– Acupuncture can be extremely helpful over the withdrawal symptoms when you give up smoking.

– Hypnotherapy works by suggesting to your subconscious mind that you won't crave cigarettes.

– Nicotine replacement therapy is available from your local pharmacy in the form of patches, gum lozenges or microtabs. They deliver a nicotine fix through your skin and can quell cravings.

– Pro-change psychology is a treatment involving one-to-one contact. According to a report in the *Journal of the American Medical Association*, treatments involving person-to-person contact are more effective when it comes to quitting.

– See Chapter 12 for more information, advice and support for quitting smoking.

7) Choose the Right Fats

A diet high in saturated fats is known to stimulate oestrogen production, which can trigger hormonal imbalance.[5] Animal products are the main source of saturated fats, so eating low-fat dairy is good to help hormonal balance in women with PCOS. At a time when you are trying to balance your hormones and remove toxins from your body, you don't want excess hormones coming from the food you eat.

What's more, if you eat too much fat your body can't excrete it as waste and you put on weight. You need to ensure that you get enough essential fatty acids, but saturated fats, found in meat, dairy products and in pies, cakes and biscuits should be avoided because they tend to be difficult for your body to digest, so they end up being stored as fat. Excess fat is thought to be responsible for the high incidence of heart disease in Western countries. So a diet low in saturated fat not only helps hormonal balance but also protects against heart disease. Here are some suggestions:

– You can cut down on meat and dairy products like cheese and milk by substituting them with fish or vegetable proteins (nuts, pulses, grains).

– You can cook with oils such as sunflower or olive rather than butter or lard.

– Full-fat milk products, butter and hard cheese are high in saturated fat and cholesterol, so choose low-fat milk, yogurts and cheeses. Milk substitutes such as rice milk, soya milk, oat milk or nut milk are also a good idea.

– Low fat is good for women with PCOS, but low fat and organic is even better. When buying dairy products, try as much as possible to buy organic to reduce your intake of chemicals and hormones. Organic dairy produce is available at most supermarkets.

8) Chemical-free Living

The amount of air pollution we breathe in is increasing and adding another layer of polluting chemicals for your body to process. 'There are over 1,000 newly synthesized compounds introduced each year, which amounts to three new chemicals a day' states the 1989 Kellogg Report. And many of these chemicals can damage your health.

It is thought that there are now over 300 chemicals which can collect in the human body, rob you of nutrients and interfere with hormonal health.[6] Since these toxins can be absorbed through the skin, you need to pay closer attention to the cosmetics you are using as well as the household chemicals surrounding you at home. If you think about the way nicotine and HRT patches work – because the drugs they contain penetrate your skin – you can see how other chemicals can make their way into your body. If you live or work in an urban or semiurban environment – as most of us do – your body is subject to a constant bombardment of chemical molecules. These molecules are in the air you breathe as well as the food you eat and the liquids you drink. They come from automobile exhausts, detergents, pesticides and so on. Their molecular structures are somewhat similar to those of oestrogen and they have the potential to occupy oestrogen receptors in your cells. This can interfere with the actual manufacture of oestrogen by the ovaries and adrenal glands, or decrease the rate of oestrogen excretion from the body, causing a build-up of the hormone. Fortunately there are many non-toxic alternatives and things you can do to protect your health:

– Use organic or all-natural products and cosmetics wherever possible. Around 60 per cent of what you put on your skin gets absorbed into your bloodstream. Natural deodorants are preferable to anti-perspirants, as sweat is the prime detoxifying process of the body and shouldn't be blocked. The aluminium in many deodorants clogs pores and stops the sweat getting out.

– Don't wrap fatty foods in clingfilm. The plastic contains toxins which can be absorbed into your food.

– Sleep with an ionizer on. Have you noticed that sea air leaves you feeling relaxed and sleepy? This is because it has more negative ions in it than normal. An ionizer is a small electrical unit that turns positive ions in your room to negative ions, helping you sleep better.

– Surround your work space and home with plants. NASA research has shown that the following plants can extract substances such as fumes and chemical cleaners, perfumes, aftershave fumes and cigarettes smoke from the air, as well as the chemicals from printers, photocopiers and VDUs: peace lilies, dwarf banana plants, spider plants, coconut palms and weeping figs, plus chrysanthemums and geraniums.

– Go for a walk in the morning, at lunchtime or in the early evening. If you work in a city, head for a park or green space. Trees give out energizing oxygen.

– Household cleaning products contain a wide variety of toxic ingredients. You can buy alternative natural products or use tried-and-true cleaners such as vinegar, baking soda and borax. Look for all-natural fresheners (see Chapter 12 for more information).

– Commonplace items in your bedroom – from alarm clock, TVs, and videos near your bed to power sockets and electric wiring – may help increase potential electromagnetic radiation exposure. Removing these possible sources of health problems is important. You could move the position of your bed away from electromagnetic objects, unplug all electrical items in your bedroom in the evening, or purchase battery-operated clocks, radios and so on.

The Pill and Your Health

The contraceptive pill is one of the most common forms of treatment for irregular periods, acne and hair loss, all symptoms of PCOS. Dianette is the brand of pill most doctors prescribe for women with PCOS, as it has anti-androgenic properties. But there is a possibility that sometimes the Pill may be doing more harm than good for women with PCOS.

It is possible that the Pill can cause a number of nutrient deficiencies. These won't affect women without PCOS as long as they eat a healthy diet, but they could make symptoms of PCOS worse, regardless of whether or not your diet is healthy. Among them are deficiencies in vitamins B_1, B_2 and B_6, causing hair loss, thinning hair and a decrease in progesterone; vitamin B_{12}, resulting in anaemia, hair loss, dry hair, brittle nails and fatigue; folic acid, resulting in skin discolouration; in the antioxidant vitamins C and E, which can cause fluctuating oestrogen levels; and zinc, which can result in acne and a decrease in oestrogen-balancing progesterone.[7]

According to the British Medical Association's *Official Guide to Medicines and Drugs*, the Pill can also affect insulin metabolism and therefore upset sugar balance and cause potential problems with diabetes: 'Oestrogens may also trigger the onset of diabetes mellitus in susceptible people, or aggravate blood-sugar control in diabetic women.'[8] Finally, some older brands of the Pill can cause oestrogen levels to soar. If your body is already fighting excess oestrogen from the environment, adding more oestrogen to the mix only compounds the problem.

You might want to explore other contraceptive methods with your doctor or healthcare provider, or other treatments for irregular periods, acne and hair loss. Or you could ensure that you make changes in your diet and lifestyle to counteract the problems that the Pill can cause. Women with PCOS who are on the Pill need

more than ever to eat a sensible diet, exercise regularly and detox
their lifestyles to avoid excess oestrogen, insulin resistance and
nutritional deficiencies. If you are on the Pill, or just coming off it,
taking a good multivitamin and mineral is a sensible idea. (For
more information about the Pill and PCOS, see Chapter 11.)

9) Stress

When we're stressed the adrenal glands prompt the release of sugar
stores into the bloodstream, triggering what is known as the 'fight or
flight' response. But instead of fighting or running away we invariably
continue fuming at our children/computer/partner, and this sugar stays
in our system, upsetting the insulin balance and making our symptoms
worse.

If you are under long-term stress, the adrenal glands become increasingly
overworked and have difficulty producing hormones in the correct
amounts.

Our bodily symptoms are bombarded with stress; over time the adrenals
start to wear down and overproduce not just cortisol and adrenaline but
testosterone as well. Excess cortisol, testosterone and adrenaline can
drive your body towards insulin resistance, weight gain, depression,
insomnia and irregular periods. Prolonged stress also increases blood
pressure. Therefore, stress-management is essential for women with
PCOS for physical and mental health.

Any stress-management regime would ideally need to act on dietary,
physical and emotional stress. You can go a long way towards reducing
your total stress by reducing your dietary stress, but you also need to
manage the emotional stress in your life, as many women with PCOS find
that their symptoms get worse under stress. This is not only due to the
stress hormones produced by the adrenals, but also because depression,
low moods and a negative mindset encourage you to feel worse and less
able to cope.

Short-term Stress

Deal with short-term stress (such as the frustration of sitting in heavy traffic) with simple relaxation techniques such as tensing your muscles hard and then relaxing them. Other techniques for short term stress include stretching regularly, deep breathing for a count of ten, talking to friends, getting a good night's sleep, drinking calming herbal teas like chamomile or lemon balm tea, having a good laugh, stroking a friendly cat or dog, or simply daydreaming about lovely, relaxing places you have been or would love to go.

Stress-management Tips

– Meditation is a great way to lower physical and mental stress. Scientists at the Medical College of Georgia, led by Vernon Barnes, studied transcendental meditation with 32 healthy middle-aged adult subjects and concluded that the technique can lower blood pressure. You may also be able to learn TM on the NHS in the UK if prescribed by your doctor for certain stress-related conditions.

– Massage can stretch tissues, increase your range of motion, help lower blood pressure and heart rate, improve breathing and be helpful in eliminating the build-up of lactic acids in muscles and waste products, because it aids blood and lymph circulation. Researchers believe that massage helps the brain produce endorphins, the chemicals that act as natural painkillers. The sense of well-being you feel from a massage can lower the amount of stress hormones such as cortisol circulating throughout your body.

– Take up yoga. MIND, the UK's leading mental health charity, recommends yoga as the single most effective stress-buster. MIND's *Guide to Yoga* followed a May 2001 survey entitled 'Exercise Your Mind', which looked into using physical exercise to control and prevent problems related to stress (for a copy of the guide, contact www.mind.org.uk).

– Think about how you react to stress. You might like to record your current stressors and rate your stress level on a scale of 1 to 10, or simply 'low', 'medium' or 'high'. Learn to recognize your body's stress signals. Common signals include: irritability, lack of concentration, mood swings, fatigue and digestive problems.

– Identify those situations and people which can trigger stress. Until you learn to cope better with stress, consider trying to avoid these triggers. You can't avoid every trigger, but you don't have to invite them into your life.

– Find ways to accept and manage any stressful situations you can't eliminate from your life completely. Don't waste energy trying to change things that can't be changed.

– Simply talking to friends, family and partners can ease stress. If you don't feel that you have anyone you can or want to talk to, a trained counsellor may help you get in touch with your feelings and give you tips on how to deal with stress.

– Try not to be a perfectionist. Let those dishes sit for a while longer, wear clothes that are comfortable, don't drive in the rush hour, return that call tomorrow.

– Set aside time to relax every day, no matter what.

– Take regular exercise to reduce stress and boost your energy. Exercise is a great detoxifier; just 10 or 20 minutes a day will help speed your metabolism and balance your hormones. It stimulates circulation, improves digestion and encourages your body to get rid of toxins. (For more information on the many benefits of exercise for women with PCOS, see Chapter 7.)

– The adrenals rely on vitamins C, B_5 and B_6, zinc and magnesium to make hormones, and these are rapidly depleted when you're stressed, so a good multivitamin and mineral every day makes sense.

10) Sleep

Not getting enough good-quality sleep makes it harder to handle stress and affects work performance, according to a poll conducted by the US National Sleep Foundation. It can also wreak havoc with your health. In addition to raising stress hormones, research findings show that sleep deprivation disrupts hormonal balance, interferes with blood-sugar levels, makes you susceptible to emotional and physical stress, causes you to age prematurely and increases the risk of diabetes, high blood pressure, obesity and memory loss.[9]

During deep sleep the body stores protein, restores energy levels and is flooded with a surge of growth hormone. Growth hormone is important for cell renewal and repair. Good-quality sleep can also help keep your blood pressure normal. Dreaming while you sleep is a way for your mind to sort through problems you are dealing with in life and get to grips with emotions so they are not stored in the body, increasing health-damaging stress levels.

Women with PCOS often get disrupted sleep caused by hormonal fluctuations. This can cause impaired reaction times, fatigue, fluctuating blood-sugar levels, depression and irritability.

How Much Sleep Do You Need?

A good night's sleep is the best tonic you can have, but it's important to realize that *quality*, not quantity, is the key. A recent study at Brigham and Women's Hospital, Boston, US, showed that a good night's sleep makes people happier, but those who had under 6 hours or over 10 hours became irritable. Seven hours seems ample for most people, but six hours of good-quality sleep beats a restless nine hours.

Are You Getting Enough Sleep?

If two or more of the items on this list apply to you, you are not getting enough good-quality sleep:

- you find waking up difficult
- you lack energy
- you need caffeine and stimulants to get you through the day
- you fall asleep often
- you yawn a lot
- you develop dark circles under your eyes.

What to Do

– Emotional factors such as anxiety or stress can interfere with sleep. Sorting out the source(s) of stress, anxiety and worry of any kind will help.

– Make sure that your bedroom isn't too noisy, light, crammed full of junk or too hot or too cold. Try not to watch TV in bed, or drink, eat or smoke before you sleep, as these are stimulants that will keep you awake.

– Lack of exercise can also lead to restlessness, but don't exercise just before you go to bed.

– Try to stick to a regular bedtime and try to keep in harmony with your internal body clock, which means you should go to bed before midnight.

– Keep fresh air circulating in your bedroom. The brain's sleep centre works better with oxygen.

– Lavender and neroli oils have sedative qualities. Try a few drops in a warm pre-bedtime bath or dropped on your pillow. The essential oils marjoram, sandalwood, rose and ylang ylang are also good for relaxation.

– Having a hot water bottle on your feet can help you sleep more soundly, according to research published in *Nature* magazine. Feet are warmer when you are in deep sleep, and speeding up the heating process can trick you into sleeping more deeply more quickly.[10]

– Use your imagination. Allow your mind to drift off to a happy memory, or imagine yourself on a warm beach, listening to the shush of the sea, smelling the suntan oil and enjoying the warmth. This will help you relax and encourage you to drift off.

– Herbal and homoeopathic sleeping remedies can help you get a good night's sleep without a hangover effect. Pharmacies and herbalists sell these – look for the valerian, hops, passionflower and Jamaican dogwood.

– Simple relaxation techniques can help. Lie on your bed and, starting with your feet and moving upwards, tense and release one muscle group at a time, ending at the shoulders, neck, head and jaw. Once your body is thoroughly relaxed, focus on slow, deep breathing. Finally repeat a phrase such as 'one', 'hum' or 'omm' and let the repetition of this sound banish all thoughts from your mind. You may actually fall asleep during this exercise.

– Massage encourages relaxation and can be an effective prelude to sleep. Try massaging a warm scented oil into your scalp and on the soles of your feet before bedtime. Or ask someone to massage your neck and shoulders for about 10 minutes.

INNER AND OUTER HEALTH

Does all the advice in this chapter mean you can never have a late night, drink unfiltered water or eat a non-organic potato again? Not at all, but remember the 80/20 rule. If you get it right 80 per cent of the time you are doing very well!

You still have to live in the real world and it is not good becoming a social hermit, as this won't make you happy in the long term. When you're out to dinner, choose sensibly, but don't punish yourself if you over-indulge a bit.

If you eat the occasional chocolate bar too many, it isn't the end of the world.

Staying up late once in a while won't harm you.

There will always be times when you eat or drink too much. Just get back on track with your healthy eating habits tomorrow.

If you read about a food that is good for you, don't go mad and eat it all the time. And don't avoid completely foods that you really crave – like chocolate, pastries or pizza. Spoiling yourself now and then will give you a lift. It is excess that is dangerous. Enjoy your food and avoid going to extremes. One chocolate bar, not ten, one cappuccino, not three, one glass of wine, not the whole bottle. You don't have to exclude everything that is naughty, just enjoy it in moderation.

Hopefully this chapter has helped you understand how much your symptoms of PCOS and general health can be improved by removing toxins from your body and your outer environment, reducing stress and getting a good night's sleep. As always, don't get carried away trying to change everything at once. Remember to take things nice and slow. Gently detoxing your diet and lifestyle isn't stressful. Sudden changes are. Life is stressful enough, don't add to it.

Assuming that you are gradually making changes by eating more healthy foods and living a more detoxed life, it's time to think about a specific eating plan which you can fit into your life. The information in Chapters 4, 5 and 7 will help you with this.

Your Sample Menu
and Recipes

So now you know the ideal way to eat – but how to go about it? Here are some ideas to help you plan the type of meals that will get you started on your diet to ease PCOS symptoms.

10-DAY SAMPLE MENU

Day One

Breakfast	Wholegrain cereal with fresh fruit, seeds and skimmed organic milk, glass of fresh-pressed apple juice
Mid-morning snack	Handful of dried fruits, seeds, nuts
Lunch	Wholemeal pitta bread filled with lean chicken and salad or hummus and salad, fresh fruit and 10 almonds
Mid-afternoon snack	Wholemeal scone with 100 per cent pure fruit spread
Dinner	Steamed fish, quorn fillet or tofu with organic brown basmati rice and stir-fried vegetables in

ginger and garlic; bowl of berries with low-fat or soy yogurt and crushed amaretto biscuits on top

Day Two

Breakfast	Sugar-free baked beans on wholegrain toast, piece of fresh fruit
Mid-morning snack	Packet of Twiglets, some dried apricots
Lunch	Big bowl of salad with tomatoes, green leaves, herbs such as basil, olives, nuts, onions, crumbling of feta cheese or other grated cheese; fruit tartlet
Mid-afternoon snack	Low-fat yogurt with chopped banana and nuts
Dinner	Mixed vegetable home-blended soup with toasted sesame and pumpkin seeds, with a veggie sausage or lean chicken/seafood sandwich

Day Three

Breakfast	Two boiled eggs with wholegrain toast, piece of fresh fruit
Mid-morning snack	Jaffa cake or digestive biscuit, herbal tea, or coffee or tea with skimmed milk
Lunch	Lean meat or fish, medium jacket potato, large helping of vegetables or salad; fruit-based dessert such as baked peaches or a crumble
Mid-afternoon snack	Vegetable sticks with low-fat cottage cheese
Dinner	Vegetable soup, 2 slices wholemeal bread with meat or fish and salad; fresh fruit

Day Four

Breakfast   1 slice wholegrain toast with cottage cheese, $1/4$ cup of blueberries and a handful of toasted almonds

Mid-morning snack   Low-fat yogurt with chopped nuts

Lunch   Carrot, orange and tomato salad, with lean meat or fish; gooseberry fool

Mid-afternoon snack   Dried fruit and packet of Twiglets

Dinner   Tofu quiche, green salad, hot fruit compôte with low-fat yogurt

Day Five

Breakfast   1 slice rye toast with caraway seeds, low-fat yogurt, glass of freshly squeezed orange juice

Mid-morning snack   Dried fruit and sesame seed crackers

Lunch   Steamed fish and vegetables, fresh fruit salad

Mid-afternoon snack   Wholemeal scone with low-fat spread

Dinner   Cajun beans topped with 1 oz of shredded cheese; baked apples stuffed with raisins and cinnamon

Day Six

Breakfast $1/2$ grapefruit, 2 whole eggs scrambled, 2 rye crisp breads

Mid-morning snack   Blueberry oat muffin

Lunch	Lentil salad with Romaine lettuce; low-fat ice-cream or frozen yogurt with chopped fruit
Mid-afternoon snack	Low-fat cottage cheese and vegetable sticks
Dinner	Wholemeal pasta, broccoli, red onion and tomato salad with lemon juice; fruit strudel

Day Seven

Breakfast	$1/2$ apple diced with granola/muesli and low-fat yogurt
Mid-morning snack	$3/4$ cup strawberries, nuts
Lunch	Vegetable fish pie, or tofu and vegetable pie, baked potato, green salad; raspberry mousse
Mid-afternoon snack	Banana and sesame seed crackers
Dinner	Fish croquettes, wholemeal rice and green beans; small bar of dark chocolate

Day Eight

Breakfast	Bowl of fruit salad topped with low-fat yogurt (or soya yogurt) and chopped nuts; glass of fresh-pressed juice
Mid-morning snack	Apple and a handful of nuts
Lunch	Hummus with wholegrain breadsticks and cucumber sticks; fruit smoothie; small bar of organic dark chocolate

Mid-afternoon snack	Two ripe apricots and a glass of skimmed or soya milk
Dinner	Roasted butternut squash (sliced in half and baked for half an hour at 200°C/400°F/Gas Mark 6); tomato, onion and chickpea stew plus a green side salad topped with walnuts; pears poached in red wine and cinnamon with a spoonful of soya cream

Day Nine

Breakfast	Slice of wholegrain toast with a teaspoon of peanut butter; small banana; fresh-pressed juice
Mid-morning snack	Bowl of cherries, handful of nuts
Lunch	Large bowl of vegetable soup and lean turkey or low-fat cheese salad sandwich
Mid-afternoon snack	Apple and one jaffa cake
Dinner	Mixed bean and vegetable casserole with wholegrain basmati rice; bowl of raspberries sprinkled with cashews and a low-fat yogurt topping

Day Ten

Breakfast	Oatmeal porridge made with skimmed milk or soya milk, with small chopped banana, half a teaspoon of cinnamon, and some berries; or Weetabix and hot milk with raisins and a half-teaspoon cinnamon
Mid-morning snack	Handful of fruit-and-nut mix

Lunch	Salad Niçoise (with tuna and hard-boiled egg); or white bean, red onion and tomato salad with garlic dressing plus a wholegrain bread roll; small strawberry tart
Mid-afternoon snack	Two rice cakes with cottage cheese and cucumber
Dinner	Thai stir-fried noodles with egg, peanuts, spring onions and vegetables or seafood; small grilled banana with two squares of chocolate grated on top

RECIPES

Sophie Elkan has PCOS herself, and has created recipes that will show you that you can create or choose dishes which aren't only good for you and easy to prepare but delicious to eat as well.

Hummus with Crudités

Serves about 4
This is a great dish as it relies on protein-packed chickpeas and fresh vitamin-filled vegetables to fill you up. It's very easy to prepare (especially if you have a hand-mixer), and also makes a good starter if you have friends for dinner, as it's not obviously 'diet' food.

1 can chickpeas in water
1–2 cloves garlic (according to taste – and how many people you may be breathing on later!)
juice of approx. $^1/_2$ lemon
tsp olive oil
tsp tahini paste
salt and pepper

Drain the chickpeas (but keep a small amount of the water). Blend to your preferred consistency. Crush the garlic and add it and the lemon juice, oil and tahini to the chickpea paste. Mix together and season.

Serve with sticks of fresh veg such as carrots, cucumber, celery and whole cherry tomatoes. It is also nice with ryvita, crackers or pitta bread.

Dahl

Serves 2–4
If you want to cut out wheat and refined carbs, this is a great lunch dish accompanied by wholegrain rice or a green salad. It's also good with grilled meat, fish or curries.

   250 g red lentils
   575 ml water
   $\frac{1}{2}$ tsp each ground turmeric, cumin and coriander
   1 tsp olive oil
   1 tblsp black mustard seeds
   1 small onion, chopped very fine
   salt and pepper
   splash of milk

Put the lentils in a small-ish saucepan. Cover with the water, add the ground spices and bring to the boil. Once boiling, reduce the heat immediately. Simmer gently until the lentils have absorbed all the water and are a soft, sludgy consistency (you may need to add more water, but do so a little at a time). Once these are cooked – usually after about 20 minutes, but do check throughout cooking because if they burn and stick to the pan it's a nightmare to wash up! – put them to one side.

Gently heat the oil and add your mustard seeds. You will need to use a pan with a lid, which should be put on as soon as the seeds are added. You will soon hear them start to 'pop' and, once you have judged that most of them have popped, add the onions and give a good stir. The mustard seeds in oil can be quite spitty, but any spitting will stop as soon as the onions are added. Cook the onions slowly to make sure they are really soft. Once they are soft enough to be eaten, add the lentil mixture and seasonings, and stir well. If your mixture is not soft enough, add milk to loosen it a little.

Tomato with Aubergine

Serves 2–4

   spray oil or no more than 1 tsp olive oil
   1 large onion, chopped quite chunky
   2 big cloves of garlic, crushed
   medium piece of cinnamon bark (or $1/2$ tsp ground cinnamon)
   $1/2$ tsp each ground/grated nutmeg, tamarind paste (if available), chilli flakes, ground cumin
   1 tsp runny honey – though not strictly necessary if you are using raisins
   handful of raisins
   1 large aubergine, diced
   $1/2$ pint of stock (chicken or veg)
   1 400-g can of tomatoes, chopped
   2 tblsp tomato puree
   salt and pepper
   sprig of rosemary (can use dried)

Gently heat the oil in a pan and add the onion and garlic. Once they have started to cook, add the cinnamon, nutmeg, tamarind paste, chilli flakes, cumin, honey and raisins. Mix well. Add the aubergine, making sure it is well covered by the spicy mixture. As the aubergine will immediately soak up the oil, add the stock to stop the pan drying out/the ingredients burning. Cook for around 5 minutes, then add the tomatoes, the tomato puree, salt, pepper and the rosemary. Stir briskly and bring to the boil. Reduce to a gentle simmer. This dish is best when it is well cooked, so if you have time it is worth leaving for as long as possible to allow the stock to reduce and thicken (this will take about an hour, but do keep checking to make sure it doesn't get dried out). Using sliced runner beans instead of aubergine is equally good.

You might like to serve this dish with a low-fat grilled halloumi cheese (available from Greek/Turkish shops and most supermarkets). If you can't get hold of any, crumble some feta over the top (Danish feta tends to be lower in fat than Greek, but the taste is not quite the same). It would also be nice with couscous or, if you are beefing up on unrefined carbs, with brown rice.

Chicken with Apricots

Serves 2–4
Similar to the dish above, this recipe uses middle-eastern inspired spices, without being at all authentic. Again it's a dish that lends itself well to being eaten with unrefined carbs.

spray oil or no more than 1 tsp olive oil
1 large onion, cut in large slices
2 cloves garlic, sliced or crushed
medium piece of cinnamon bark (or $1/2$ teaspoon of ground cinnamon)
$1/2$ tsp each ground/grated nutmeg, tamarind paste (if available), chilli flakes, ground cumin
handful of sliced almonds (optional)
fresh chicken cut in small chunks (1 breast per person)
$1/2$ pint of stock (chicken or veg)
2 handfuls of dried apricots, chopped, best to use sulphur-free
large carrots, sliced on the diagonal (at least one carrot per person)
3 tblsp tomato puree
sprig of rosemary (can use dried)
salt and pepper
fresh coriander leaves as an optional garnish

Gently heat the oil in a pan and add the onion and garlic. Once they have started to cook, add in the cinnamon, nutmeg, tamarind, chilli flakes and almond, if using. Mix well. Add the chicken and cook quickly to 'brown' all the pieces. (Add a bit of stock if needed to lubricate the pan.) Now add in the chopped apricots and carrots and stir to make sure all ingredients are evenly dispersed. Cook for about 5 minutes. Once carrots start to soften, add the tomato puree, rosemary, salt and pepper and finally the stock. Stir well and bring to the boil. Cover and reduce to a low simmer. Leave for around 20 minutes.

When you return check the carrots to see if they are soft and ready to eat. Once they are, remove the lid and reduce the stock to a gravy consistency. Serve with coriander, if available/desired.

Tropical Fruit Loaf

   300 g wholemeal plain flour
   1½ tsp baking powder – or just use self-raising flour
   175 g muscovado sugar
   1 tsp grated lime rind
   1 egg
   1 medium banana – mashed (this is a good way of using up very ripe bananas that you wouldn't want to eat if you're fussy like me!)
   1 tub low-fat fromage frais or 0 per cent fat Greek yogurt
   2 handfuls of raisins
   25 g dessicated coconut

Heat oven to 180°C/350°F/Gas Mark 4 and prepare a loaf tin with butter and flour or greaseproof paper.

Add the wholemeal flour to a mixing bowl (with baking powder if needed) and stir in the sugar and lime rind. Make a well in the middle of the mixture and add the rest of the ingredients. Stir really well and spoon into your loaf tin. Put in the oven for about 40 minutes – it may need a bit longer, so make sure you check the centre is cooked before you take it from the oven.

You could ice this with a glaze made of icing sugar with a little hot water and lime juice added to blend it to a sauce-like consistency, or even sprinkle the top with demerara sugar before you put it in the oven – though I myself don't bother, as I like to think of it as 'guilt-free' as possible!

Cheat's Brulée

The soft fruit in this one could include bananas, berries, melon or peaches, or you could gently cook a little apple, pear or rhubarb (just place in a pan on a low heat and leave to stew down in their own juices – though you may have to add a tiny bit of water just to set it off. You could even add a little booze – whiskey, brandy, amaretto – but that would not be so virtuous!).

fruit of your choice
1 tub 0 per cent fat Greek yogurt/low-fat fromage frais
demerara sugar

Line the bottom of a ramekin with your fruit (about 1-inch deep). You may like to add some spices such as ground cinnamon or clove, or just leave it quite simple. Add your yogurt to fill the ramekin to the top and generously sprinkle with sugar. Whack under a pre-heated grill until the sugar bubbles.

Sophie Elkan's Cheat's Risotto

Fantastic comfort food and quick and easy to prepare.

Serves 2–4
1 tsp olive oil
medium onion, chopped fine
garlic (optional)
for seafood, $^1/_2$ tsp chilli flakes, juice of about $^1/_2$ lemon and a tsp of thyme
for veg or chicken, try oregano or basil with a little nutmeg
your choice of content – prawns/seafood, chicken or veg: mushrooms, asparagus, broad beans
250 g risotto rice
2 tblsp tomato puree or 1 tub of 0 per cent fat yogurt, depending on whether your soul is crying out for creamy comfort food or more robust redness

575 ml stock (chicken or veg, or Spanish 'paella' sauce if you can find it)
grated low-fat cheese (optional but really helps)

Gently heat the oil in a deep pan and add your onions, garlic and spices
(if using). Cook for about 5 minutes, then add your choice of ingredients
in order of the amount of time they will take to cook – for example, if you
are using raw chicken, add that first until it has browned, then add the
veg. Give it a good stir, then add the risotto rice. Season well and, if using
tomato puree, add this in now. Give it a good stir, then add the stock.

Bring back to the boil. Once boiling, give a vigorous stir, and cover
immediately. Turn the heat down as low as it will go and leave for 15
minutes. Do not remove lid during this time. Once the time has elapsed,
remove the lid – the rice should be cooked. If not you will need to add a
little more liquid and keep an eye on it. If you are using yogurt for a
creamy risotto, add it now. Stir and add cheese if desired. Allow to stand
and cool for a couple of minutes, sprinkle with a little parmesan cheese
if you like, and serve.

'Easy Conscience' Vegetable Curry

This is a real 'comfort' treat that is incredibly low fat and nutritionally
fantastic, with lots of those amazing and varied vegetables. Protein is
somewhat lacking in this meal, but is present in the yogurt, nuts and the
lentils if you choose to include them.

Serves 2–4
    2 onions
    garlic cloves (as many as you like)
    5 sprays of 'fry light' or no more than 1 tsp olive oil
    4 white cardamom pods
    2 cloves
    2 bay leaves
    small piece of cinnamon bark (or $1/2$–1 tsp ground cinnamon)
    1 tsp fresh coriander (or $1/2$–1 tsp ground coriander)
    1 tsp cumin seeds (or $1/2$–1 tsp ground cumin)

small nub of chopped fresh ginger (or $1/2$ tsp ground ginger)
$1/2$–1 tsp each ground turmeric and chilli flakes (or ground chilli)
handful of peanuts/chopped walnuts/cashews or chopped Brazil nuts
$1/2$–1 pint stock
1 medium-sized potato, diced
2 sweet potatoes, diced
4 medium carrots, sliced thick
any other vegetables you may have: broad beans, baby
sweetcorn/frozen sweetcorn, peas, mushrooms, cabbage, sugar snap
peas or mangetout, cauliflower, etc.
a good squeeze of tomato puree
1 tsp mango chutney
handful of lentils (optional)
small pot of total 0 per cent fat Greek yogurt
coriander as garnish if desired

Finely chop onions, crush garlic and start to sauté in heated, oiled pan.
Stir constantly and add the spices and the nuts. Once the aroma starts to
be released and your onions start to go translucent, add the powdered
spices. If the pan is sticking add a little water or stock. Add the potato and
sweet potatoes to the spicy mixture, stirring constantly. Let these soften
for about 5 minutes, then add the carrots. Add some stock or water and
let this mixture cook for around 5 to 10 minutes.

Add the rest of your vegetables and stir together. Add the tomato puree,
mango chutney and the lentils (uncooked) if you are using them; give a
good stir. Add enough stock to more or less cover the vegetables and
bring to the boil. Once boiling cover, and immediately reduce the heat.
Stir occasionally and check after 15–20 minutes to see if veg are nearly
cooked. Once you feel that they are cooked to your liking, take the lid off
to allow the sauce to reduce. Once the consistency is as you like, remove
from the heat and allow to cool slightly. Add the yogurt. If you have any
fresh coriander you could use this to garnish.

This is quite a filling, starchy dish. If lentils have been added it should be
sufficient as a one-pot dinner. However, you can serve it with a number of

things depending on your mood. It works with plain, steamed basmati rice. Wholewheat chapattis are also good. Another favourite is to have with poppadoms (great if you are trying to be wheat-free, as they are made with gram flour). You can buy uncooked poppadoms and put them in the microwave, with no oil, for just under a minute. Keep an eye on them, as they will puff up quickly and can easily burn.

Liver-boosting Potato and Vegetable Salad

This detoxifying recipe has been adapted from Dr Sandra Cabot's Liver Cleansing Diet program. For more information, see Chapter 12.

> 10 small new potatoes with skins on
> black pepper
> sea salt
> 1/4 tsp paprika
> 2 tblsp cold-pressed olive oil
> 2 cups broccoli
> 6 cups washed lettuce, dried and torn into small pieces
> 2 cups chopped spinach
> 1 cup alfalfa sprouts
> 1 cup finely sliced red cabbage
> 1/2 cup low-fat mayonnaise

Boil the potatoes for approximately 20 minutes until tender. Drain, cool and cut into chunks. Place in a bowl. Add pepper and salt, paprika and oil and toss well. Place potato mixture on baking paper and bake on the top shelf of a pre-heated oven set at 190°C/375°F/Gas Mark 5 for 10 minutes.

Steam the broccoli for 5 minutes or until tender. Remove from heat and plunge into very cold water for approximately 40 seconds to prevent overcooking, then drain well.

Place the lettuce and spinach in a bowl, add the sprouts and cabbage. Cut broccoli lengthwise and add to greens. Add the low-fat mayonnaise. Remove potatoes from the oven and add to the salad.

MIND MEAL RECIPES

The MIND Meal

The MIND Meal is one practical example of how food can be used to lift mood. The mental health charity MIND have drawn up a list of foods thought to have either a positive or negative effect on mood. Launched by MIND in 2000, the resulting MIND Meal contains foods which are thought to make you feel better and think more clearly. MIND continues to receive positive feedback from people who have tried and tested this menu.

The MIND Meal consists of the following three courses:

1 Wheat-free pasta with pesto and oil-rich fish
2 Avocado salad and seeds
3 Fruit and oatcakes for dessert.

What the MIND Meal *doesn't* include is just as important as what it *does*. You won't find artificial additives, added sugars or stimulants like coffee, nor foods which can trigger allergies such as wheat and milk. What the meal does provide are foods containing valuable vitamins and essential fats – important for emotional and mental health. The oil-rich fish, as well as providing vital Omega-3 essential fatty acids, is also a source of tryptophan. Tryptophan is the essential 'good mood protein' which is also found in avocado, seeds, dried apricots and walnuts. Absorption of the tryptophan is assisted by the carbohydrates contained in the dessert. The tryptophan is converted into the mood-enhancing brain chemical serotonin, and the banana and avocado also provide some-ready made serotonin. Because the meal has a medium to low GI, it will provide a slow release of energy to keep you feeling good for longer. To recap on GI or get a list of other low-GI foods, see Chapter 2.

The recipe below serves two hungry or up to four not-so-hungry people. Preparation time shouldn't be more than 30 minutes, and all the ingredients should be available from your local supermarket or health food store.

Wheat-free Pasta with Pesto and Oil-rich Fish

250 g/9 oz packet of wheat-free pasta such as corn and vegetable pasta shells
100 g/4 oz pesto sauce
170 g/6 oz tin salmon or other oil-rich fish such as mackerel, herring, sardines, pilchards in brine oil or spring water or fresh tuna (canning reduces tuna's Omega-3 content)

Cook the pasta in boiling water per the instructions on the packet. When the pasta is ready, drain and transfer to a warmed serving dish. Add approx. 1 tablespoon pesto sauce per person and gently mix in with the pasta.

Open the tin of fish, drain liquid, remove or crush any large bones and flake with a fork. Add to the pasta and pesto and mix gently together.

Avocado Salad and Seeds

250 g/8 oz bag mixed lettuce or 80 g/4 oz bag watercress
1 avocado
handful (25 g/1 oz/1/4 cup) sunflower seeds
handful pumpkin seeds

Place the mixed salad in a serving dish. Remove the skin and stone from the avocado, cut into small pieces and add to your mixed salad. Sprinkle on the seeds.

Serve plain or with olive oil or the salad dressing of your choice.

Fruit and Oatcakes Dessert

2 bananas
2 apples
8 dried apricots
8–12 oatcakes
40 g/2 oz/1/2 cup (broken) walnuts

Peel the bananas and rinse the apples and dried apricots. Remove the apple core, cut all the fruit into small pieces and place in a small saucepan. Add a minimum of 3 tablespoons of water and simmer gently for 10 minutes or until the fruit is soft, adding more water to prevent the mixture becoming too dry and sticking to the pan.

Arrange the oatcakes in the bottom of individual dessert bowls (you may have to break them to make them fit).

When the fruit is soft, pour over the oatcakes. If the fruit mixture contains enough liquid, the juices will soak into and soften the oatcakes.

Serve with a sprinkling of broken walnuts.

Part Two

TACKLING YOUR PROBLEMS

Fine-tuning Your Diet to Beat PCOS Symptoms

Not everyone with PCOS is the same. Eating a basic healthy diet, doing the gentle lifestyle detox and working out which type of food combinations or regime suits you best will help to keep you in optimum health now and protect your health for the future. But if you have a particular symptom or health problem along with PCOS, this can be a cause for special concern or focus. In this chapter we'll show you how you can add in adjustments, supplements and power foods, either on their own or with other natural medicines, to help you beat your particular symptoms.

SAFETY FIRST

Herbal Medicine

Only use herbs under the care of a health care practitioner who is familiar with herbal medicine. Inform your doctor about all other medicines and herbal preparations you're taking. If you have a history of cardiovascular disease, diabetes or glaucoma, or you are pregnant, use herbs and supplements from your nutritionist or medical herbalist only in consultation with your doctor.

Natural Therapies

Make sure that you are working with a skilled and qualified practitioner, and always let your doctor know what you are doing. Ideally your doctor can recommend a practitioner.

For more advice and information on all the supplements, herbs and natural therapies mentioned in this chapter, see Chapter 8. Chapter 12 is also a good source of information.

Finding the Diet-boosters that Could Help

For PCOS and Acne   see below
For PCOS and Fatigue   see page 123
For PCOS and Irregular Periods   see page 127
For PCOS and Depression   see page 130
For PCOS and Fertility Problems   see page 139
For PCOS and Excess Hair   see page 152
For PCOS and Hair Loss   see page 153

PCOS AND ACNE

Acne isn't necessarily something you grow out of. Recent studies show that up to 50 per cent of adults between the ages of 20 and 40 have some form of acne. In one study, over 80 per cent of women who were referred to a dermatology clinic for acne were found to have PCO/S. This is not to say that all women with PCOS have acne – the figure is thought to be around 30 to 40 per cent.

I always thought I would eventually grow out of acne, but I'm in my thirties and I still get acne. It's embarrassing and sometimes quite painful. People do their best to pretend they haven't noticed but I know they have. They probably think I don't wash, or that I eat lots of junk food or something. The truth is my diet is very healthy and because my face gets so oily I have to wash it several times a day.
Melanie, 36

According to Anthony Chu, senior dermatologist at the Imperial College of Science, Technology and Medicine, Hammersmith Hospital in London, the cause of acne isn't chocolate, fatty foods, cakes or sweets, although sometimes they can make the condition worse, nor poor hygiene, which again will aggravate the problem. The cause is thought to be an increase in the skin's oil production. This oil, called *sebum*, is made by the sebaceous glands in the skin, which react to the male hormone testosterone. Even though many women with PCOS have slightly higher levels of testosterone in their bloodstream, some women with acne have no more than usual. So it seems that women with PCOS who also have acne have sebaceous glands that are extra-sensitive even to normal levels of testosterone. Once the excess oil blocks the pores it can form blackheads and attract bacteria. Pus can then collect at the site as white blood cells rush to fight off the infection.

You can buy creams, gels and treatments for acne from your pharmacy. Check with your pharmacist to get the right one for your skin type. For women with PCOS who have acne, the usual treatment is the contraceptive pill for at least six months. This is because it has anti-androgenic effects which can help to prevent sebaceous glands being triggered to produce more oil (see Chapter 7 for more information about oral contraceptives). Your doctor may also prescribe antibiotic creams or pill to reduce the number of bacteria on your skin and calm inflammation.

✤ Heavy makeup can block pores and exacerbate infections. Keep makeup to a minimum, and cleanse thoroughly with a mild (not astringent) skin-care product. Never leave makeup on at night, and choose oil-free moisturizers and makeup. Opt for loose rather than pressed powders, and powder blushes instead of creams. Look for the word 'non-comedogenic' on labels.

✤ Always try to cleanse your skin twice a day, but don't use harsh cleansers or toners with alcohol – these strip the skin of natural oils, encouraging it to produce more in response.

✤ Avoid abrasive scrubs. They do remove dead skin, but they can cause irritation and make acne worse. Use one specifically recommended by a dermatologist if you use one at all.

❀ Never pick or squeeze spots – this can cause scarring.

❀ Choose oil-free sunscreens in gel or liquid form for your face rather than a cream or a lotion, and avoid other products, such as cold cream, which can block your pores.

❀ When your acne eventually clears – and for many women it eventually does – your skin may be drier than usual. You will need to use a lighter moisturizer.

❀ Bear in mind that any skin type can have PCOS acne: dry, oily or combination. Use products that are designed for your skin type, complemented by diet, exercise and medicines to reduce the acne. Exercise is important because it encourages a healthy blood flow to your face, which can help flush out toxins. It also reduces the amount of free androgens in the bloodstream – one of the triggers of PCOS acne.

Dietary Strategies

Although acne isn't caused by a poor diet, a poor diet will have an impact on your whole body and make acne worse. A good balanced diet is therefore important, and certain food choices are beneficial. Try to follow the diet laid out in Chapter 2; in addition, here are a few helpful tips:

Eat a diet high in fibre to rid the body of toxins.

Sulphur-rich foods such as eggs, onion and garlic are thought to be helpful for skin conditions. Carrot juice is full of skin-nourishing nutrients, as are cabbage, watercress, spinach and parsley juice. You can also take sulphur supplements.

Eat foods rich in zinc, including shellfish, soybeans and sunflower seeds, and a small amount of raw nuts. Zinc is an antibacterial agent and a necessary element in the oil-producing glands of the skin. A diet low in zinc may promote flare-ups.

Ensure an adequate intake of the antioxidant vitamins A, C and E, which are important for healthy skin tone. Debate rages about whether or not vitamin C in any form can actually penetrate the skin. However, some women have found vitamin C creams useful for acne. Taking vitamin E can improve skin elasticity. Dabbing vitamin E oil on acne and scars can help them to heal. Pierce a capsule of vitamin E with a pin and squeeze the oil out to apply it. If you suffer primarily from blackheads, retinol, a vitamin A derivative, softens and expels them and can help to prevent the inflamed red spots later on.

Make sure you get your EFAs. Flaxseed oil and primrose oil are good sources of the essential fatty acids needed to keep skin smooth and clear and to repair damaged skin cells.

Eat 'live yogurt' containing *bifidus* and *acidophilus* bacteria every day. This will help rebalance the bacteria in your gut so that your skin is protected against inflammation. The yogurt can be eaten on its own, flavoured with chopped or pureed fruit, poured onto fruit or cereal or swirled into soups or casseroles.

Limit your intake of alcohol, sugar, processed food, iodized salt, butter, caffeine, chocolate, eggs, fried foods, spicy foods, meat, margarine, wheat, soft drinks and food containing hydrogenated vegetable oils.

Garlic is a powerful antibiotic. Grate it in your food or take a supplement every day. This will also help to protect your heart.

Natural Therapies

✼ A study conducted by the Department of Dermatology of the Royal Prince Alfred Hospital in New South Wales, Australia found a 5 per cent solution of tea tree oil was as effective as a 5 per cent solution of benzoyl peroxide for most cases of acne, and had no side-effects. Use a tea tree moisturizer.

✼ Kombucha tea, which has antibacterial and immune-boosting qualities, has been found by many people to be beneficial for acne. Dab it on or drink it.

✼ Pure aloe vera gel is antibacterial and soothing. Some women with PCOS have reported big improvements from dabbing the pure gel on their acne every day. It is also renowned for healing burned skin and scars, so can be put to good use on old acne sites on the skin as well.

✼ For angry and inflamed acne, witch hazel is cooling and soothing. Dab directly on the acne.

✼ Echinacea is one of nature's most powerful antibiotics. Dab a tincture or cream on the affected skin daily.

✤ Ketsugo is made from isolutrol, a substance originally derived from shark's bile, but now synthesized. It is rich in antioxidants and, according to Dr David Fenton of St John's Department of Dermatology at St Thomas' Hospital in London, it appears to be able to regulate the production of sebum and soften the skin.

✤ Burdock root and red clover are powerful blood-cleansers. Milk thistle aids the liver in cleansing the blood. A medical herbalist may prescribe these for you. Other beneficial herbs include alfalfa, cayenne, dandelion root, saw palmetto, agnus castus and yellow dock root. All these should be prescribed by a medical herbalist.

✤ If your acne is severe, don't use steam treatments. They can make the condition worse. If the condition is mild to moderate, lavender, red clover and strawberry leaves can be used to steam sauna the face for antibacterial protection.

✤ The homoeopathic remedy pulsatilla is for acne which is worse at puberty and before menstruation. Kali brom is for itchy pimples on the face, chest and shoulders brought about by hormonal changes. If you aren't sure about a homoeopathic remedy straight from the shelf, consult a practitioner.

✤ Light therapy, which involves shining different types of light on the acne, from UV to simply coloured light, can help. Red lights have been shown to open capillaries and boost circulation, while blue light has the opposite effect. Ask a dermatologist about it.

I remember starting my period at age 13; by 15 my face was covered in acne. It was so horrible I wanted to die. I never got hair on my face. I guess there wasn't any room for it! I also stopped having periods when I was 20. I went to the doctor and she found a lot of cysts in my ovaries. She recommended the birth control pill to regularize my periods and clear my acne.

I didn't want to go on the Pill. I'd tried it once and it made me feel sick. I read a magazine article about naturopathy, so instead saw a naturopath who recommended a wholefood diet, with natural supplements like agnus castus and aloe vera cream, a good multivitamin and mineral supplement, and a regular exercise programme. The results came very fast. My hair started to shine again, my spots got better and I stopped feeling so darn tired all the time. I still get the odd flare-up of acne, but nothing like the eruptions I used

to get. *About a year later my periods started again. I was thrilled. Ironic isn't it? I used to dread having periods. They were inconvenient. Now I'm delighted to have them back. They make me feel as if I'm normal.*
Miranda, 28

PCOS AND FATIGUE

Although doctors don't yet recognize fatigue (or lack of energy) as a symptom of PCOS, many women with the condition say that they feel tired a lot of the time and need to sleep for longer hours. It can be hard to wake up and get going.

I need a good 10 hours' sleep, and if I can I'll nap in the afternoon too. It's the only way for me to keep going. I'm on medication for PCOS and my mum thinks that is making me feel so tired, but I'm not so sure. Before I was put on the medication I did notice that I wasn't as energetic as I used to be. It's especially bad when I have my period. I'm just exhausted.
Nicola, 31

Some mornings the alarm clock goes off I turn over and go straight back to sleep. It's not like me; I always used to love the mornings. These days I really haven't got half the energy I used to have. I'm not sure if it is my PCOS or age that is slowing me down so much.
Beverley, 40

Fatigue can be caused by a dip in blood sugar, especially overnight when the body is fasting and blood-sugar levels are low. Insulin resistance may also play a part in creating tiredness. Another factor that needs to be taken into consideration is the idea of 'unopposed oestrogen' (see page 12).

Maintaining a regular menstrual cycle by managing PCOS with self-help measures such as diet and exercise could help to get rid of your fatigue. The best thing you can do to regularize your period is eat a healthy, hormone-regulating diet according to the guidelines in Chapter 2. It's especially important for a healthy menstrual cycle that you get your essential fatty acids, B vitamins and zinc, and to reduce caffeine and alcohol consumption. You can also work on reducing your stress levels (we all know that worrying about a late period can delay it even more), get sufficient rest and maintain a healthy body weight, neither under- nor overweight. Also you should try to stop, or at least cut down, on smoking. It's well known that smoking can inhibit ovulation.

Do bear in mind that fatigue can also be linked to emotional factors like depression. When you feel low your energy is often sapped and feelings of listlessness and tiredness can take over. Wanting to stay in bed and sleep a lot is one of the signs of depression. If you think this may have something to do with your tiredness, read the section below on depression and go and see your doctor.

Other conditions to rule out with your doctor include thyroid problems, anaemia, vitamin and mineral deficiencies, food intolerances, allergies and post-viral syndrome, all of which can lower energy levels.

Dietary Strategies

Diet has a big part to play in keeping energy levels constant, periods regular and avoiding slumps – usually in the mid-morning and mid-afternoon. We've said it before and we'll say it again: plenty of fresh fruits and vegetables, wholegrains such as brown rice and wholemeal bread, and proteins such as soya, pulses, fish and lean (preferably organic) meat can all help. Avoid energy-robbers such as sugar, alcohol, fats, caffeine, white-flour products and highly processed foods.

Eating raw foods is thought to boost energy levels. The argument is that over-cooking can destroy essential nutrients. Keep cooking to a minimum. Most foods only need to be simmered or steamed lightly. This doesn't mean you can't eat cooked foods, it just means you should balance them with raw ones. One of the best ways to achieve this balance is to drink fruit and vegetable juices or 'smoothies' on a daily basis. All you need is a vegetable peeler, a sharp knife and cutting board and, of course, a juice extractor. For sustained energy throughout the day, experiment with a variety of fruit and vegetable juices as an addition to your daily diet.

Juiced-up Ideas

❋ The most basic juice cocktail is carrot and apple. Combine 4 carrots with 1 apple.

❋ Apple and spinach is an amazing combination for cleansing the digestive tract, improving elimination and boosting energy. Try 3 apples combined with a handful of spinach and drink twice a day – especially important before bedtime.

❋ For a smoothie booster – add three handfuls of berries to one apple, a banana, a teaspoon of cold-pressed hempseed oil and a sliver of tofu. Blend and shake.

Key energy-boosting nutrients include beta carotene, vitamin D, E and K, calcium and zinc, but the most important energy foods are those rich in B complex group of vitamins, which comprise vitamin B_1, B_2, B_3, B_5, B_6, B_9 (folic acid), B_{12} and biotin. These are found in abundance in wholegrains such as millet, buckwheat, rye and quinoa (a South American grain that is becoming more readily available), corn, alfalfa and barley. If these grains are sprouted their energy quotient is increased many times, as the enzyme action involved in the sprouting process increases their nutrient value. Sprouting is the process of soaking then germinating the seed and finally eating the growing live sprouts or sprinkling them on salads, adding them to juices, etc. The full range of B vitamins is also to be found in fresh, green vegetables.

Other nutrients essential for energy production:

Vitamin C	found in fruit and vegetables such as oranges, potatoes and peppers
Magnesium	green vegetables, nuts and seeds
Iron	plentiful in grains, pumpkin seeds and lentils

Copper	part of the make up of Brazil nuts, oats, salmon and mushrooms
Co-enzyme Q10	found in beef, sardines, spinach and peanuts
Spirulina	an excellent protein energy-giving source. Take 4 spirulina tablets a day, or add 4 tablespoons of powder to a smoothie.

Sunflower oil and sunflower seeds are packed with essential fatty acids, vitamins E, A, D and B complex, the minerals zinc, iron, calcium, manganese, potassium. They're an excellent source of protein, too, making them one of the finest energy pick-me-ups, especially when combined with some dried or fresh fruits as a snack.

Wild blue green algae contains virtually every nutrient known to man. It can provide a feeling of well-being, vigour and vitality. You can get supplements in health stores.

Sea vegetables or seaweed are a highly digestible source of minerals. They can improve digestion and enhance mental energy.

Flax seeds (also known as linseeds) and hempseeds are the most abundant source of Omega-3 and Omega-6 fatty acids in perfect balance. They can help regulate weight and bowel function, lower cholesterol, enhance skin tone and improve immunity and reproduction.

Ginseng is of the most use for people convalescing or under major stress. Supplementing with ginseng needs to be considered on an individual basis with a qualified practitioner, as there are different types. Korean ginseng is the most stimulating, so exercise caution if you have high blood pressure or oestrogen-related hormonal problems. All types will be beneficial if the lack of energy is stress related.

Natural Therapies

❋ Get a good night's sleep.

❋ Start a gentle exercise routine. Even a 10-minute daily walk around the block can be energizing.

❋ If you are overweight, start to lose weight gradually (see Chapter 7). Keep your sense of humour well stimulated. Spend more time with people who make you laugh, watch favourite comedies on TV or video, go to a pantomime even if you are grown up.

❋ Sign up for some voluntary work to help people with a problem or cause you feel strongly about.

❋ Dance or listen to upbeat music.

❋ Keep your creative powers well stimulated. Play thinking games, read a good book, take up a new interest or hobby, learn a new language, join a debating society or enrol in an evening class.

❋ Lime essential oil, lemon or peppermint in your morning bath can invigorate you.

❋ A cup of peppermint or lemon or ginger tea can help you feel more refreshed and awake.

❋ Experiment with therapies which are thought to boost energy: acupuncture, shiatsu, aromatherapy, yoga and massage.

PCOS AND IRREGULAR PERIODS

I haven't had any periods for four years. You'd think I'd be glad, but I'm not. It just doesn't feel right. The only way I can describe it is like constipation – and that's pretty unpleasant – or you want to sneeze and you can't. I feel uncomfortable and unnatural.
Tracy, 24

I had always had irregular periods – sometimes going for months without – and then my husband was diagnosed with high blood pressure. His doctor told him that he really needed to start eating more healthily to reduce the risk of heart disease. I started to make changes to our diet immediately. Within three months his blood pressure fell, and my periods came like clockwork.
Lynn, 37

One of the most common symptoms of PCOS is irregular or absent menstruation. It is also one of the most worrying. Regular menstruation signifies good health and fertility. Absent or irregular bleeds are a sign of poor health and hormonal dysfunction, typically thyroid problems or PCOS. Your doctor will probably put you on the Pill to regulate your cycle, but it is important to point out that Pill bleeds are not 'real' periods. They are simply withdrawal bleeds from the effects of the Pill.

In order for you to have a normal menstrual cycle where ovulation occurs, you need an oestrogen-progesterone balance. Many things can cause an imbalance of oestrogen and progesterone. In addition to PCOS, poor eating habits, wild swings in weight, eating a lot of processed carbohydrates, and very low-fat diets which deprive the body of the good fats needed to stay healthy and manufacture hormones will all affect hormonal health. Studies show that stress can also be a major problem and leave its mark on the menstrual cycle.[1]

If you have PCOS and don't ovulate for several months, your ovaries' secretion of oestrogen becomes erratic due to the hormonal imbalance created by your condition. You may have surges of the hormone, which cause erratic, heavy and painful bleeds. Oestrogen and progesterone are intended to balance each other and work in harmony for maximum hormonal health. When the protective effect of progesterone is lost, symptoms like weight gain, depression, loss of libido, water retention and fatigue can begin to take hold.

If you don't want to go on the Pill, either because it doesn't agree with you or you want to regularize your periods in order to get pregnant, there are many things you can do to help yourself:

First and foremost, eat a healthy diet according to the guidelines in Chapter 2.
Take a multivitamin and mineral that includes B vitamins, zinc, vitamin C, beta carotene and vitamin E.
Maintain a healthy body weight (see Chapter 7).

Natural Therapies

❈ Massage your abdomen with lavender or melissa oil (if periods are irregular), rose or cypress oil (if periods are heavy), marjoram oil (if your periods are painful). Use a total of 2 drops of essential oil in a teaspoon of carrier oil for massage, up to 4 drops in the bath.

❈ If you suffer from period pain, try a warm bath with a couple of drops of geranium (mood-lifting), chamomile (painkilling) and clary sage (muscle relaxant) oils to ease cramping and soothe pain. You could also try the good old hot water bottle. Willow bark tablets are natural alternatives to aspirin and are available from health food stores and herbalists. The homoeopathic remedies lachesis (for pains that improve once bleeding starts), arsenicum alb (for pains accompanied with chills and fatigue) or belladonna (for labour-like pains with gushing red blood flow). Take the remedy that suits your symptoms in the 30c potency. If the relief is only temporary, repeat up to twice more at 45-minute intervals. For heavy periods try ipecac (if you have backache) kali carb (if you have fluid retention and feel washed out) or belladonna. Take as for painful periods.

❈ The homoeopathic remedies graphites or actaea racemosa are often prescribed for irregular periods, but each woman is unique and remedies should only be prescribed by a homoeopath on an individual basis. The exception is a missed period resulting from sudden emotional shock, when you can try aconite 30c twice a day for two to three days. If there is no relief after a week, see a practitioner.

❈ If your periods have stopped completely or your ovulation pattern is irregular, the herbal remedy agnus castus can be helpful. Other useful herbs include false unicorn root, blue cohosh, wild yam, dong quai, dandelion, liquorice, motherwort, siberian ginseng, and squaw vine. Raspberry leaf tea can also help tone the pelvic area and improve circulation. You would need to see a herbalist for an individual prescription.

Studies have shown that acupuncture can be very effective at relieving pain and regulating the hormonal system. Yoga can also restore hormonal balance and there are specific exercises to ease tension in the lower abdomen. Deep breathing and stretching can help relax your muscles and your mind and increase the blood flow to the pelvic region.

Progesterone Creams

If your periods are irregular or you get a very heavy bleed, you might want to try natural progesterone cream to balance and regulate your cycle. The progesterone is absorbed into the fatty layer beneath your skin and then taken into your bloodstream. If you are not having periods at all you need to apply the cream daily for several months to feel an effect. If you have irregular periods, you need to use the cream for three weeks out of every four. If your periods are very heavy, confine the cream to the second half of your menstrual cycle.

You can get progesterone cream on prescription from your doctor in the UK; in the US it is readily available (see Chapter 12). It's important to work with your doctor if you want to use natural progesterone cream. It is called 'natural' but it is still a drug, and until studies prove otherwise its use remains controversial. Too much of any hormone can have the opposite effect from the one desired.

PCOS AND DEPRESSION

Many women with PCOS do get depressed, stressed or anxious. Being diagnosed with PCOS can be a frightening experience. Fear about health and fertility issues, and the reality of living with a chronic illness, can mingle with resentment that your symptoms and condition were misdiagnosed and misunderstood for so long. In addition, symptoms such as acne and weight gain can make you feel less feminine and bring up feelings of insecurity about your body.

I hated the way my body started to look. I had bad acne and hair on my chin. I didn't have a waistline anymore, as I was gaining a lot of weight. I didn't want to look in a mirror unless I was plucking out hairs or caring for

my spots. I felt so unfeminine and unattractive. Looking back, I can see that I was heading for a nervous breakdown.
Sasha, 44

I was convinced I'd never have children and I'd be fat for the rest of my life. I got seriously depressed. Why was this happening to me? I didn't deserve to have PCOS.
Anna, 29

We don't know yet if depression is a symptom of PCOS or whether the PCOS symptoms such as weight gain and infertility cause depression. It can sometimes be impossible to know which came first. Many experts do agree that our physiology, which is closely linked to hormonal fluctuations, is an important key to understanding depression, and that hormones influence every aspect of our lives in ways that aren't yet fully understood.

Don't forget, though, that there are also other types of depression which may have nothing to do with your PCOS, such as post-natal depression, reactive depression after the loss of a job, the ending of a relationship or a bereavement, seasonal affective disorder (brought on by a lack of natural sunlight) or biochemicial depression (a result of a chemical imbalance in the body, sometimes due to a nutritional deficiency or an inherited predisposition). Some people also experience depression as a result of an allergic reaction or food intolerance, the most common being to wheat and dairy products.

Depression, stress and anxiety can manifest themselves in physical symptoms such as insomnia, headaches, fatigue, sudden loss of or increase in appetite, emotional symptoms such as feelings of sadness, hopelessness, emptiness or guilt, and behavioural changes such as poor concentration, loss of libido, memory loss and withdrawal from social interactions.

Everybody, whether they have PCOS or not, gets low from time to time, but if you feel that you are not coping and this isn't just a low mood, make sure you seek professional advice from your doctor (see Chapter 12 for contact details of helpful and informative organizations).

Help from Your Doctor

Depression can be treated many ways. Often, talking treatments or cognitive behavioural therapy with a professional counsellor can help. Prescription antidepressants are also frequently used to treat depression. Prozac is the most talked-about antidepressant, but there are many other antidepressants which your doctor may prescribe you, along with instructions on how much to take and for how long. There are no specific antidepressants used for women with PCOS; it is likely that you and your doctor will have to experiment with various medications before you find what works best for you.

Your attitude plays an important role. A woman with a negative attitude towards PCOS will often feel depressed. A negative attitude is often a forerunner of stress and depression. First and foremost you need to believe that you can control your condition and improve your health. Equally important is physical well-being. If your diet is poor, your body is stressed and you won't be able to respond well to the challenges life throws at you. As a result you will be more susceptible to infections, you are unlikely to make healthy food choices, and you will feel much worse.

In addition to a healthy diet, a consistent programme of physical activity can contribute to a sense of well-being. We'll discuss the mood-enhancing powers of exercise in more detail in Chapter 7.

Self-help to Lift Your Mood

✺ Refocus negative thoughts to positive ones. Talk positively to yourself and make an effort to stop negative thinking. Remember: PCOS has not destroyed your health. Your health and well-being are in your hands.

✺ Set some goals. Achievement, even if it is small, is vital for tackling low moods. But be realistic. Start small, with things like giving yourself a proper lunch-break every day, throwing out clothes you never wear anymore, calling your mother every week. You will feel lighter at heart when you start to cross things off your 'To Do' list.

❊ Plan to have at least 30 minutes of gentle exercise every day.

❊ Plan to eat a healthy diet.

❊ Make an effort to reach out to others, but make sure you take care of your own needs too.

❊ Pamper yourself with treats such as an aromatherapy massage or a hot bath, a facial at a salon or in your bathroom, a new haircut, a night out with friends, a walk in the park, a day at the coast. These things can make us feel so much better, but we never seem to do them enough.

❊ Use relaxation techniques (massage, guided imagery, breathwork, prayer, yoga). Experiment until you find the right technique or techniques for you.

❊ Music can have powerful effects on mood and may help you feel better, especially if you can sing or dance along.

❊ Take time for personal interests, hobbies and vacations.

❊ Stress-management classes can help reduce tensions. In the UK, Boots run free stress-management programmes as part of their 'Happy Life Skills' sessions.

❊ Have a good cry. Letting out pent-up emotions can leave you feeling calmer and better able to deal with the situation at hand.

❊ Have a good laugh. Laughter sends chemicals called endorphins whizzing around your body to make you feel naturally high. So do something to get you chuckling, from watching a funny film to calling an old friend.

❊ Encourage family and friends to support and help you.

❊ Peer support: VERITY is a UK-based PCOS support and information service. The Polycystic Ovarian Syndrome Association (PCOSA) is a US-based support and education organization for women with PCOS. Sharing your experiences with others and knowing you are not alone can lighten the load. (See Chapter 12 for more information.)

Dietary Strategies

Within the brain, chemicals help transmit messages from one nerve cell to another. Two such substances – serotonin and norepinephrine – are endorphins that seem to affect our moods. The body makes these endorphins from the food you eat; therefore you can to a certain extent raise the level of these substances in your brain by eating specific foods.

The main sources of endorphins are sugary and carbohydrate-rich foods. This is why you may feel happier when you have eaten a bar of chocolate, a cake, biscuit, white bread with jam or rice pudding. The problem is, as you know, that the sudden influx of sugar leads not just to a rush in serotonin but a rush of insulin, too. Insulin breaks down the sugar, quickly leading to a drop in both sugar and endorphin levels. This leaves you feeling even lower than you did before.

To avoid blood-sugar swings, it's best to eat a healthy meal soon after you have eaten a sugary treat, or that you choose to get your sugar/endorphin fix from a more slowly absorbed carbohydrate. Good examples include a wholemeal biscuit or wholegrain bread with a topping of fresh fruit or a low-sugar fruit spread. Having a little fibre intertwined with your sugar helps to lift the low, but not too fast, so you stay happy for longer. Swap sugary refined carbs for unrefined ones, such as fruit, wholegrains and veg – these all take longer to digest and so there isn't such a rapid increase in blood sugar. You might also want to take supplements of chromium and vitamin B_3, both of which help regulate blood sugar.

Serotonin and norepinephrine are also made from tryptophan and L-phenylalanine, amino acids present in certain protein foods. Some experts suggest that we take supplements of endorphin-producing amino acids, but this can lead to stomach upsets and diarrhoea unless you follow a personalized prescription from a nutritional therapist. The best way to avoid exposing yourself to a lack of serotonin and norepinephrine is to eat a healthy, varied and balanced diet, like the one outlined in Chapter 2.

If you feel that your depression may be due to a nutrient deficiency, arrange to see your doctor for a few blood tests.

Deficiencies of the B vitamins and vitamin C are most commonly associated with depression. It's a chicken-and-egg situation: Deficiencies can lead to a low mood, but a low mood can also lead to lethargy and lack of interest in preparing good food.

A zinc deficiency has been noted in some people with depression. This mineral is also essential for healthy reproductive function. Other mineral deficiencies likely to cause depression are iron, potassium and magnesium. Depression has also been linked to a deficiency in essential fatty acids.

Nutrient	Good Food Sources
Vitamin B	Dairy produce (milk, yogurt, cheese, butter), eggs, fish, wholegrain cereals and wheatgerm, dark green vegetables such as broccoli, asparagus, spinach, yeast extract (e.g. Marmite), nuts (such as Brazil nuts and walnuts), beans, wheatgerm, fresh orange juice and bananas. Folic acid, a B vitamin, is found in green leafy vegetables (such as spinach) and legumes
Vitamin C	Oranges, strawberries, kiwis, grapefruit, lemons, citrus fruits, blackcurrants, rosehips, melon, papaya, spinach, Brussels sprouts, cabbage, leafy greens, cauliflower, red and green peppers, tomato juice, potatoes, green peas and asparagus
Zinc	Shellfish (such as oysters, mussels, crab and lobster), canned sardines, turkey, lean red meats (such as lamb), hard or crumbly cheese (such as Cheshire), wholegrain cereals
Iron	Spinach, egg yolks and oily fish
Potassium	Potatoes, bananas, orange juice, tomato juice, dried apricots and prunes, and natural yogurt
Magnesium	Wholemeal and granary bread, leafy green vegetables, milk, yogurt, meat, apricots and bananas

EFAs   Oily fish, leafy green vegetables and oils (such as
              flaxseed oil)

Anaemia

Symptoms of iron deficiency (anaemia) include tiredness,
irritability, pallor and a general feeling of being run down. Severe
iron deficiency can lead to breathlessness, headaches and an
inability to complete simple tasks. If you have any of these
symptoms, see your doctor to check the cause. It's important that
you know which kind of anaemia you have. Iron-deficiency
anaemia is relatively easy to correct through changing the foods
you eat and making lifestyle changes, but the other kinds of
anaemia are a little trickier and you should consult your doctor.

The two most important nutrients involved in iron-deficiency
anaemia are iron and vitamin C. Vitamin C helps your body absorb
iron. You should therefore concentrate on having plenty of the
foods mentioned above.

Some Foods to Lift Your Mood

These are all foods rich in mood-boosting carbs plus essential vitamins
and minerals.

Leek and potato soup
Carrot and orange soup
Warm goat's cheese salad
Chicken with melon, grapes and asparagus
Smoked cheese and wholemeal pasta
Oysters with cream and parmesan
Spicy fish kebabs
Prawn curry
Coconut chicken
Sausage and bean casserole
Mixed fruit with butterscotch sauce

Wholemeal fruit scone
Flapjacks
Date and walnut cake
Brazil nuts
Shellfish, especially crab
Banana cake
Lemon cake
Toast with banana

Strange as it may seem, many investigators have found that garlic not only has positive effects on blood and cholesterol but that garlic-eaters also experience a decided lift in mood. Hot chilli peppers can produce a similar effect.

(See page 111 for a comforting, mood-lifting recipe from UK mental health charity MIND.)

Melvin Konner MD of Emory University, Atlanta, US, notes that new studies on brain physiology supports caffeine's use as a mild antidepressant. He sees nothing wrong with using caffeine in this way if the depression is mild and does not need medical attention. However, as pointed out earlier, for women with PCOS too much caffeine can wreck your mood, disturb your sleep and rob you of essential nutrients. If you can't live without caffeine, try to stick to no more than one or two cups of tea or coffee a day.

Some studies suggest that chocolate can influence serotonin levels, but you're unlikely to eat enough to make much difference, according to Dr Peter Rogers, a psychologist at the University of Bristol. Chocolate probably boosts mood because from an early age we've viewed it as a treat. Again, it's best to eat chocolate only once in a while, but really enjoy it when you do.

In addition to eating healthy foods that can lift your mood, you might benefit from the gentle detox advice given in Chapter 3. Internal pollution can contribute to a low mood; flushing out toxins from your body with lots of fruit and vegetable juices and raw foods may be able to shift depression.

A month after my 30th birthday I was diagnosed with PCOS. Acute depression hit me from out of nowhere. This was nothing like the depression I had known in the past when my sister died. This wasn't about grieving or loss or the blues. It was a depression that hit me physically as well as emotionally. I felt like I was being suffocated. At its most intense I couldn't even go into work.

My mother was very concerned and suggested I visit a medical herbalist. The herbalist put me on progesterone cream and vitamin E. The black moods went and, feeling more optimistic again, I started to exercise regularly and eat healthily. My periods are completely normal, my acne is improving and I'm confident that I can manage my PCOS.
Paula, 32

Natural Therapies

St John's Wort

There are many brands of St John's Wort (*Hypericum perforatum*) on the market which can vary in strength and potency. An overview of 23 clinical trials into St John's Wort and depression was carried out by Klaus Linde and colleagues and published in the *British Medical Journal*, declaring Hypericum extracts to be 'significantly superior' to placebo and indeed, 'similarly effective' to standard antidepressants. Reported side-effects include nausea and extra skin sensitivity but, unlike many antidepressant drugs, St John's Wort has not been found to lower sex drive or impair the ability to experience orgasm.

A dose of 900 mg of an extract of St John's Wort daily has been shown by studies to be effective in counteracting mild depression. However, over-the-counter preparations contain only 300 mg of extract. Visiting a registered medical herbalist for a tailor-made prescription is one way to make sure you are getting the correct dose. For more information see Chapter 8.

In addition to St John's Wort, other herbs thought to relieve depression include:

❈ ginger
❈ gingko biloba
❈ liquorice root
❈ oat straw
❈ peppermint
❈ lemon balm
❈ Siberian ginseng

A medical herbalist can tell you how to take these.

Homoeopathy can also be helpful in cases of mild depression. Again, you'd want to consult a qualified practitioner.

PCOS AND FERTILITY PROBLEMS

Irregular periods, weight problems, acne, facial hair – I had all the classic symptoms of PCOS and was diagnosed when I was 26. I was told that getting pregnant wouldn't be that easy, but here I am 10 years later with three healthy kids. When I was 28 I visited a naturopath and she put me on a special fertility-boosting diet. Not only did my acne clear, but I got pregnant three months later. I'm very lucky because PCOS can put the brakes on fertility and it could have been so very different for me.
Sue, 38

Infertility is when you cannot have a baby. If you have PCOS you are not infertile, there is just a possibility that you may have problems getting pregnant, something called sub-fertility.

Doctors won't tend to investigate a couple for fertility problems for at least a year, or possibly two if they are younger than 30. This is because many 'normal' women and healthy couples can take at least a year to get pregnant anyway.

To conceive you need to ovulate, and for women with PCOS we know that this doesn't always happen. If your periods are irregular it is likely that you are not ovulating – or that if you are, you cannot predict when you will be.

In a normal 28-day cycle, ovulation occurs around 14 days after the first day of your period. There is some variation around this; most doctors agree that the fertile week could run from day 10 to day 17 of a 28-day cycle. If your cycle is 26 days, your fertile week would be days 8 to 15; if your cycle is 32 days long, your fertile week would shift to days 14 to 21.

Most doctors and specialists recommend that couples trying to conceive should make love every day or at least every other day over their fertile week. This is fine if you have a regular cycle, but what happens if your cycle isn't regular or you aren't menstruating at all? If you're not willing to wait one or two years before looking for help, what can you do?

Study after study show that conceiving and pregnancy outcomes are improved if both you and your partner are in good health. Remember, fertility isn't just a woman's problem. (Of couples who go to fertility clinics, roughly one-third are found to have problems relating to the woman, one-third the man and one-third are combined problems or unexplained ones). The better the health of both partners, the more likely conception, the less likely generic and chromosomal defects and the better the chance that the pregnancy will proceed normally. Even if you aren't ovulating and eventually need medical treatment, the better your health and that of your partner, the better the likely outcome.

A poor diet, as well as too much stress, can lead to nutritional deficiencies, hormonal imbalances and irregular periods. For proof of this, think back to a time when you were really upset or anxious about something – you probably skipped a period or your period came late.

Research is proving that a high percentage of women diagnosed with infertility have nutrient deficiencies.[2] Without enough zinc, vitamin A and magnesium, for instance, your sex hormones can't even be produced, let alone function. These substances are needed at every stage of the reproductive process.

A basic, healthy diet should be the first step in starting to help yourself and your partner. It may take several months for this to have an effect. Ideally, you should both start a healthy eating plan about six months before you actually start to try to conceive. Not only will this maximize your chances of a regular cycle and ovulation, but there is another benefit as well: Some experts believe that what you eat prior to conception is just as significant as what you eat during pregnancy for the health of the baby-to-be. The egg is a product of your diet and, according to Irwin Emanuel, MD, Professor of Epidemiology and Pediatrics at the University of Washington in Seattle, 'There are very good data to show that foetal growth affects adult disease risks. If you are undernourished your baby could well become "programmed" at conception to develop high blood pressure, clotting disorders, abnormal glucose, insulin and cholesterol problems and even hormonal problems like PCOS.'

Dietary Strategies

For optimum fertility and the health of the unborn child, a healthy, nutritious diet is extremely important. Your diet should follow the guidelines outlined in Chapter 2. See also the tips on eating to regularize your periods on page 127.

Dietary fats should not be neglected. If you don't eat enough fat, hormone production will be compromised. A diet too low in fat can cause fertility problems. It is true that some fats should be avoided because they are high in calories and increase the risk of infertility – these tend to be saturated fats from red meats and full-fat dairy products. But unsaturated fats, such as those found in seafood, soya beans and lean meats, have many health benefits.

Especially important for women trying to conceive are the essential fatty acids. For hormonal regulation you need a diet rich in Omega-3 and Omega-6 food sources. Flaxseed oil, sea vegetables, green vegetables and cold-water fish are rich sources of Omega-3. Unrefined vegetable such as like sunflower, soy and olive oils, as well as green leafy vegetables, are rich food sources of Omega-6.

I never imagined I'd have a problem, but when we started trying for a baby my periods stopped. I was prescribed Clomid, followed later by IUI treatment, where sperm is injected directly into the womb. I didn't get pregnant. It was devastating. Even more upsetting were the mood swings and excessive hair now growing on my face, tummy and around my nipples. I felt like I should be in a freak show. I had an X-ray and was diagnosed with PCOS. I longed for a baby and decided that IVF was our last chance. Three attempts failed. I was devastated and depressed. I started to comfort-eat and the weight piled on.

Eventually I decided to stop having the treatments and try a diet and lifestyle detox. I bought a book published by Foresight [see Chapter 12] and tried to follow the guidelines as best as I could. I didn't really believe it would work, but I thought I had nothing to lose.

After six months I'd lost weight and felt so full of energy. I was ready to try IVF one more time. I felt so much more hopeful this time. The IVF worked! I gave birth to a healthy baby boy. It was our dream come true, we had waited so long. Then something amazing happened a year later – I got pregnant again without IVF. It was the most incredible, amazing miracle.
Jill, 37

I spent most of my twenties feeling ugly, not knowing that I had PCOS. My spots were horrible and I'd been trying to treat them since the age of 13. They got worse as I got older, and none of the therapies I had tried worked. I wasn't overweight but I was very self-conscious about my body. I felt ugly inside. I didn't make the links between my irregular periods, acne and facial hair until a friend read an article and showed it to me. I went to see my doctor and a scan confirmed PCOS. I was given hormone-based tablets, but they gave me terrible headaches so I stopped taking them.

I saw a dermatologist, who helped me control my acne. She also recommended regular exercise along with some simple dietary changes. I was also advised to take the herb milk thistle to encourage the blood flow to my skin and clear out toxins. After keeping to her regime for 18 months, I fell pregnant. My doctor had told me I would need fertility treatment to conceive,

*and that gaining weight with pregnancy would make my symptoms worse,
but this wasn't the case for me. I proved him wrong. I visited a medical
herbalist, who prescribed agnus castus and also suggested that I start
exercising regularly and taking a multivitamin and mineral, an essential fatty
acid and an antioxidant complex supplement. Much to my surprise, my
symptoms seemed to vanish. I now have three healthy, happy children, my
cycles are like clockwork, I'm not overweight, my acne is under control and I
feel good about myself.*
Deborah, 33

Fertility-boosting Supplements

There are so many things you can't control about your fertility, but diet,
at least, is not one of them. Research has shown that remarkable
improvements in fertility can result from doses of the fertility-enhancing
vitamins and minerals listed below. However, always consult a
nutritionist, because self-prescription won't give you the best
combination for you. Always remember that too much, even of a good
supplement, is bad unless it's combined with a healthy diet.

If in doubt, perhaps the safest cause of action is to take a daily
multivitamin pill, as a study carried out at Leeds University in the UK has
shown that women with fertility problems are twice as likely to conceive
if they take a multivitamin and mineral pill every day.

Supplement	Found in
Folic acid	Spinach, green beans, Brussels sprouts, milk and fruit. Arguably the most important supplement you should be taking. Every woman thinking about having children should ensure she takes a folic acid supplement of 4 mg every day. Folic acid-deficiency is associated with neural tube defects in babies-to-be
B vitamins	Wheatgerm, wholegrain products, yeast extract and brown rice – particularly crucial for women who drink large amounts of coffee. It is advisable to take B vitamins in complex form rather than individually

Vitamin B_2	Yogurt, yeast, eggs, green leafy vegetables, mushrooms, fruits and cereals
Vitamin B_3	Lean meat, fish, peanuts, bran and beans
Vitamin B_{12}	Fish, meat, eggs, milk and cheese. Vitamin B_{12} is especially important for vegans and vegetarians
Vitamin C	Raw fruits and vegetables
Vitamin D	Your requirement for this nutrient increases dramatically should you get pregnant
Vitamin E	Wholegrains, vegetable oils, seeds, nuts and green leafy vegetables
Calcium	Dairy products, fish, nuts and dried fruits
Essential fatty acids	Evening primrose oil, olive oil, flaxseed oil, oily fish, avocados, sunflower and sesame seeds
Iron	Eggs, fish, dried milk, dark green vegetables. Your requirement for this nutrient increases once you get pregnant
Manganese	Wholegrains, nuts, onions
Magnesium	Milk, nuts, seafood, wholegrains
Selenium	Herring, tuna, whole wheat, broccoli, garlic
Zinc	Seafood, milk, whole-grains and dried fruit

Antioxidants can counter the negative effects of free radicals – molecular fragments which can cause damage to your fertility and your body. Ensuring an adequate intake of the antioxidant vitamins and minerals can be extremely beneficial. The most important food-derived antioxidants are beta carotene (the non-toxic part of vitamin A), vitamins C and E, as well as certain B compounds and the minerals selenium, manganese, copper and zinc.

Preventable Risks

It is sensible to tackle dependency on anything known to inhibit fertility – alcohol, smoking, caffeine, drugs and overeating – and to try to avoid polluted areas and too much stress.

Studies show that women are drinking more than ever before, especially the young and career-minded. Any woman with PCOS who drinks heavily reduces her chances of fertility and doubles her risk of miscarriage or having a baby with a deformity. The risks start to rise at the equivalent of four measures of spirits or glasses of wine, or two pints of beer or cider per day, increasing steeply at about three times these amounts. The alcohol-related risk is greater if you are over the age of 35, use the contraceptive pill, smoke and your diet is poor.

Drugs alter the chemistry of your body; you should always check with a medical expert before taking any form of medication. This includes over-the-counter remedies and alternative therapies. Street drugs such as ecstasy, cocaine and heroin are known to reduce fertility and increase the risk of miscarriage. If you have PCOS, tell your doctor that you are concerned about your fertility so that you know all the options available to you.

Smoking is a well-known inhibitor of fertility. Many women smoke because they think it keeps their weight down, but it is possible to stop smoking and not put on weight. Books on quitting smoking can offer support and ideas, or you may prefer to ask your doctor's advice.

Too much caffeine may also prove to be harmful, because caffeine depletes the body of essential nutrients. The Food Standards Agency (FSA) has warned that excess caffeine could lead to miscarriage and suggests that expectant mothers consume no more than 300 mg of caffeine a day – the equivalent of four cups of coffee – following new research linking excessive caffeine consumption to low birthweight babies and miscarriages. The advice given by the Royal College of Midwives is that 'Caffeine intake during pregnancy in moderation is perfectly safe,' but the key word here is *moderation*. Try to limit your intake of tea, cola, coffee and chocolate to a sensible amount.

Weight, in particular body fat, has a direct influence on egg production and can be the cause of a woman's inability to conceive. Women who are too heavy – or too thin – can experience fertility problems.

Losing weight made all the difference. I lost nearly a stone and was pregnant within a month. I couldn't believe it. I've got PCOS and thought I didn't stand a chance, but my doctor urged me to lose the weight. It was absolutely the right thing to do.
Pat, 40

Excess weight can affect ovulation, as fat cells produce oestrogen, and too much oestrogen prevents the egg from being released. Oestrogen is also the main ingredient of some contraceptive pills. Obesity can also affect insulin levels in women, which can cause ovaries to overproduce male hormones and stop releasing eggs. Studies show that regardless of the infertility diagnosis weight loss in overweight women improves fertility.

Low weight or dramatic weight loss can lead to a temporary weakening of an important hormonal message which the brain sends the ovaries. In some cases eggs may be produced and released, but the lining of the uterus is not ready to receive the fertilized egg. In other cases, ovulation simply does not occur. If your body weight drops too low your periods will stop.[3]

Eating a healthy, balanced diet should ensure that you stay at a healthy body weight. Erratic eating habits, dieting and weight fluctuations can all damage fertility. After years of yo-yo dieting and weight gain and loss, many women, regardless of whether or not they have PCOS, do experience problems with their fertility. If you have PCOS and are dieting to lose weight it is vital that you ensure your body is getting all the nutrients it needs to maintain ovulation and healthy reproductive function. In Chapter 7 we'll discuss weight loss, exercise and maintaining a healthy body weight in more detail.

Avoiding pollution and harmful radiation may also be beneficial. Unfortunately, in this modern world these are difficult to avoid. Metals and chemicals are found in a wide range of items, including tooth fillings, detergents, pesticides and plastic packaging and drinking water. Some metals, particularly lead and cadmium, have been linked to studies with fertility problem of all kinds.

Ways to avoid pollution include:

- ❄ Filter drinking and cooking water.
- ❄ Eat organic produce – not just fruit and vegetables but also pulses, seeds, dairy produce.
- ❄ Avoid unnecessary exposure to chemicals.
- ❄ Avoid smokey atmospheres and places where there are traffic fumes.
- ❄ Avoid food wrapped in plastic, aluminium or tin. Store food in china or glass rather than plastic and cook with cast iron, stainless steel or enamel pans rather than aluminium.
- ❄ Keep microwaving to a minimum, and make sure your oven is safe.

(For more tips, see Chapter 3.)

Another way to improve your fertility is to take regular exercise, as long as this is not taken to extremes. Too much exercise can have a disastrous effect on fertility, because it can stop ovulation occurring. But a moderate amount of exercise is beneficial. It doesn't have to be strenuous, but do try to get out of breath, as this is good for the heart and lungs. Try around 30 minutes at least two or three times a week. Swimming and walking are recommended.

More and more these days we are hearing about celebrities or career women who are slowing down the pace of their lives to try and have a baby. According to studies from the University of Utrecht in Holland, women who delay giving birth to concentrate on their careers should be told how falling fertility levels in their late thirties can make it harder to get pregnant in the future, whether they have PCOS or not. It's impossible to generalize, but it does seem that there is a connection between infertility, delaying childbearing and a demanding, hectic lifestyle with no time for relaxation.

DIY Fertility Tests

If you are in your thirties and putting off children for the future, there are tests you can take which may tell you more about your chances of getting pregnant later in life. Initially you should consult your doctor or a fertility specialist. If you are considering such tests, bear in mind that, because they are only related to the cycle previous to your last, these tests may not be the reliable or accurate predictors of fertility they claim to be.

Dr Gill Lockwood, Director of Midland Fertility Services in the UK, has pioneered a fertility MOT for women which measures hormone levels that indicate if the ovaries are slowing down. 'There is nothing worse than being in an infertility clinic with a successful 30-year-old woman for whom time has run out and hear her say, "If only I had known there could be a problem." '

The London medical firm Genosis claims to have developed the world's first fertility kit. The kit has been devised as an early warning sign for couples trying to conceive. It's said to be able to tell men in 40 minutes and women in 15 whether they are able to have children and whether it is advisable to postpone pregnancy any further. The female test measures levels of hormones secreted by the ovaries and also the 'shelf life' of the number of eggs stored there – a low egg count means a greater likelihood of infertility.

Stress-reduction is important for optimal health. Stress occurs when there is an imbalance between the demands of your life and your ability to cope with them. Constant stress over a long period of time will upset hormonal balance, deplete the body's resources, cause anxiety and depression, diminish the immune system and inhibit fertility. We need a certain amount of stress and challenge in our lives, but it should be a positive kind of stress, not stress that damages our health. Negative stress should be avoided or, if it can't be, we need to learn how to deal with it in a positive way.

One way to cope better with the stresses in your life is to ensure that you are in good health by eating right and exercising regularly. For other stress-management tips, see Chapter 3.

Natural Therapies

Alongside the dietary changes mentioned in this book, you may find it helpful to try some complementary approaches such as herbal medicine, acupuncture, aromatherapy, reflexology or homoeopathy. The herbal remedies listed below have proved to be effective in balancing hormones and boosting female fertility. For more information, see Chapter 8.

Warning: If you have PCOS and are trying to get pregnant, it is essential you consult a good herbalist or health professional with experience in using herbs so that the remedies can be tailored to your individual needs.

Agnus Castus
This herb can stimulate progesterone production and help regulate your cycle. In one study, 48 women diagnosed with infertility took agnus castus daily for three months. Seven of them became pregnant during that time, and 25 of them started to menstruate regularly. If your periods are irregular, it might be worth trying this herb over a few months – ideally using a prescription from a medical herbalist.

Dong Quai
This is used for menstrual problems in traditional Chinese medicine. It is a well-known tonic for female reproductive system. It can help with absent periods and regulate irregular periods.

False Unicorn Root
This North American herb has a balancing effect on hormones. Mixed with other herbs it is often given to women with PCOS to regulate periods.

Acupuncture

Acupuncture has proved to be successful in boosting fertility according to various studies.

According to researchers Gerhard and F Postneck at the University of Heidelberg, 45 infertile women who received acupuncture had more pregnancies than those in a control group. It can correct hormonal imbalances and problems like PCOS and endometriosis. The acupuncturist would concentrate on regulating your menstrual cycle and strengthening kidney function.

Reflexology

Reflexology can also aid conception by releasing unblocked energies into the body.

Homoeopathy

In homoeopathy, every woman with PCOS will be given a different remedy because each person is treated according to their individual constitution. Having said that, Pulsatilla is often given for women with no periods or irregular periods. Because infertility is so complex, it is better to consult a qualified homoeopath so that treatment can be individualized. Specific help can be given for PCOS (see Chapter 12 for advice on how to contact a homoeopathic practitioner).

Aromatherapy

This natural treatment utilizes the therapeutic properties of essential oils, extracted from flowers, leaves, stem backs or wood of aromatic plants and trees. Essential oils can be extremely potent concentrates. They can be absorbed into the bloodstream via the skin, hair and lungs (through inhaling). Oils in the bloodstream will circulate for several hours, while those inhaled will stimulate the limbic system in the brain which deals with emotion. In massage, tiny amounts of essential oils would be mixed with other base oils such as almond. Oils of particular relevance to helping with infertility problems are:

Clary sage   a tonic for the womb and hormone balancer
Geranium   regulates the hormonal system
Jasmine   a hormone-balancing as well as a nerve-calming oil
Melissa   helps regulate your periods and lift your spirits
Rose   helps regulate your periods and promote self-confidence
Ylang ylang   a hormone-balancer and womb tonic.

Pre-conceptual Care

Ruth Delman, co-founder of the Chi Health Centre in London, advocates pre-conceptual care to boost fertility. 'Herbs and acupuncture can assist ovulation,' she says 'but alleviating the pressure to conceive can also make a huge difference.' Julie Gerland is a clinical hypnotherapist who specializes in emotional clearing, which she believes is necessary for parenting. 'Subconscious worries can prevent conception, so hypnotherapy can deal with doubts about your future role as a mother,' says Julie.

There can be a huge pressure these days on women to have it all: the body, the job, the partner and the baby. It is assumed that this is what most women want, but you may have your doubts and insecurities about motherhood and feel pressurized by those around you to conceive. This pressure isn't the encouraging force it is intended to be, and can sometimes make conception a stressful business. If you do think you want a baby it is important that you find out if this is what you *really* want, and not what those around you expect.

Back to Basics

Eating well won't guarantee fertility, but it will increase your chances. As leading nutritional therapist Marilyn Glenville points out, even if you do eventually need medical intervention, 'a healthy diet will increase your chance of success'. With assisted conception treatments and techniques it is still important that you are as healthy as possible.

Many women who want to start a family learn a lot about ovulation and fertility treatments, but forget the simple things they can do to improve their chances of conceiving. And the best self-help strategy, which has the backing of scientific research, is to eat a healthy diet.

PCOS AND EXCESS HAIR (HIRSUTISM)

Hirsutism is the medical term for an excess of facial and body hair in women. Androgens determine the type and distribution of the hairs on your body, and hair grows in androgen-sensitive places – that is, areas in which men are prone to grow hair, such as on the face, the midline of the chest around the nipples, the abdomen and the lower back.

About 60 per cent of women with PCOS show hirsutism, varying from growth of some coarse hair on the upper lip and chin to excessive coarse hair on the face, trunk and thigh. Hirsutism is not a challenge to health itself, but for many women it causes serious problems in their social life, threatening their self-esteem and affecting their quality of life.[4]
Gabor T Kovacs, PCOS specialist at Monash Medical School, Box Hill Hospital, Melbourne, Australia

What I wouldn't give to have one day without shaving, plucking or feeling self-conscious about my facial hair. I never go anywhere without my hand mirror and razor. I'm a school teacher and children can be very cruel. I live in fear of the day I get caught without shaving. Having hair in places ladies aren't supposed to have hair has inhibited me as a woman. I lack confidence with men and I'm ashamed of my body.
Sally, 30

Not all women with PCOS have hirsutism, but many do. 'Along with irregular periods it is one of the most common symptoms, and at times the most distressing,' says Dr James Douglas, reproductive endocrinologist at the Plano Medical Center in Plano, Texas, who treats women with PCOS.

Studies show that, with a healthy diet and weight loss, symptoms of PCOS such as hirsutism decrease.[5] Exercise can also improve hirsutism, because the fitter you become the lower your body fat and the better your insulin and glucose control. This in turn reduces the amount of testosterone produced in your ovaries and the amount of testosterone circulating in your bloodstream. If you are spending too much time plucking and waxing and shaving, in addition to your basic healthy diet you may want to seek advice from your doctor for hormone therapy. The contraceptive pill is the most usual medical way to tackle the problem of excess hair. A new drug called Vaniqua, approved by the FDA (Food & Drug Administration) in the US, is also now available as a cream.

Natural Therapies

The most common herb used specifically for excess hair in women is saw palmetto, although it's important to remember that it is best taken in combination with other herbs and prescribed by a qualified medical herbalist. Saw palmetto is used mainly to treat prostate problems in men due to its effect on reducing androgens, so it is also thought to be useful in the treatment of excessive hair growth in women.

I had a terrible time when I was growing up. You know how much your peers can make you feel inadequate. Not only was I overweight, I was hairy as well. Nobody wanted to sit with me. Taking saw palmetto really helped me stop feeling and looking so hairy. I feel much more confident as a result. Thank God I've found something that actually works for me.
Nina, 26

PCOS AND HAIR LOSS

Otherwise known as *alopecia*, hair loss can be one of the symptoms of PCOS. There are many types of alopecia, some resulting in total baldness, but this is not what women with PCOS get – if this is your problem, it has not been caused by PCOS.

Women with PCOS get a gradual overall thinning of the hair, or thinning at the corners above the temple. Hair gradually goes see-through – the sort of hair that appears as a fine fuzzy halo when a light shines on it. This is called *alopecia androgenetica* and is the female version of male-pattern baldness. Remember, though, it is normal to lose around a hundred hairs a day. If you think you are losing more than this, then you probably have alopecia.

I had no idea how important my hair was to me until I started losing it. I used to have thick, glossy long brown hair. Suddenly my hair was thin, dull and damaged. I'd also noticed that I was losing a lot more hairs every time I brushed it or washed it. I knew that hair loss could be one of the symptoms of PCOS, but my doctor didn't seem that concerned. I was really scared.
Jo, 34

Dr David Fenton, Consultant Dermatologist at St Thomas's Hospital, London, says, 'Women with PCOS can get hair loss and thinning due to excess androgens in the bloodstream. Mostly women with PCOS first notice thinning on the top of the head, but the shedding may be variable due to when ovulation occurs and when it doesn't.' Dr Fenton believes that the contraceptive pill can cause an increased shedding of hair, though he does say that this often evens out as the body adjusts to the new hormonal balance and new hair growth-cycles can begin.

Dietary Strategies

Balancing out hormonal cycles in PCOS through eating a healthy diet is the best way to tackle the problem, regardless of whether you take the Pill or any other medication on top.

Hair loss can be made worse by nutritional deficiencies, especially a lack of iron, vitamin B_1, vitamin C, vitamin E, zinc or lysine (an amino acid). Follow the diet recommendations in this book.

Make sure you don't go short on essential fats and water. Dry hair that lacks shine and breaks easily is often a sign of lack of EFAs.

Since hair is 98 per cent protein, make sure you are eating enough lean fish and poultry. Try to avoid sugar and sugary products. Include in your diet foods which are rich in biotin, and use hair-care products containing biotin. Good food sources include brewer's yeast, brown rice, green peas, lentils, oats, soybeans, sunflower seeds and walnuts.

Avoid foods containing raw eggs. Raw eggs not only pose the risk of salmonella but are high in avidin, a protein that prevents biotin being absorbed. Cooked eggs are fine.

The grain alfalfa, particularly in its sprouted form, has long been believed to stimulate hair growth.

Iron deficiency can cause hair loss, so consider bumping up the amount of iron-rich foods you eat from lean organic meats to apricots, dark green and dark red vegetables.

Try not to eat too many cereal grains or soya products if you are losing hair, as these contain substances called phytates which can cause deficiency in minerals such as calcium, iron and zinc. Under normal dietary circumstances this wouldn't cause a problem, but it could if you overdo the cereal grains and the soya. Once again, moderation is the key.

I couldn't lose weight no matter what I tried. Every time I forgot about calories for a minute I'd put on weight, which of course I then couldn't lose. I went to a dietician who put me on a very low-fat diet. I got so tired so I quit. I tried other low-fat diets, but by now I was beginning to get moody fits and lack of concentration. I even thought that on top of my PCOS I had some adult attention-deficit disorder. This went on for nearly a year. I started out worrying about my weight, but that was not my main worry now. I'm a driving instructor and I need to be able to concentrate. I was also losing my hair.

At first the loss was hardly noticeable – a few extra hairs on my comb or brush. Within a couple of months, though, there were a lot more.

A friend of mine suggested I go to a dietician who had helped her lose weight. I was sceptical at first and thought it would be very humiliating, but the first few sessions weren't about slimming and weight-loss goals but about basic nutrition. I was surprised at how little I knew. What really helped me was learning about a healthy diet and how eating too little fat could not only cause irregular periods but skin and hair problems and lack of concentration. My dietician suggested I keep a food diary to see how balanced my diet was.

I began to see that all I was eating was sugar, sugar, sugar. Even the complex carbs I had were fast-acting or high GI with no fat or protein to slow down the insulin response. I started to combine my carbohydrates with moderate amounts of protein and fat. For example, eating a handful of nuts with my salad or eating some natural peanut butter on my fruit.

I also began to read up about portion sizes. Mine were way too big. One helpful tip I picked up was to 'eyeball' my portions – to have meat or fish portions the size of a deck of cards, and starchy foods that are no bigger than a tennis ball. Also that there should always be three times as many vegetables as starchy foods. With practice, making visual estimates became second nature and were very helpful, especially when eating out. In less than a month my hair loss started to ease and I got my powers of concentration back at work. In fewer than three months I started to lose weight and feel attractive for the first time in years.

Jo, 34

Natural Therapies

❀ Scalp massage (easy when you are shampooing your hair) can be useful, especially combined with essential oils. Scottish researchers have found that 44 per cent of alopecia patients who massaged their heads daily with a mix of thyme, lavender, tea tree and cedarwood oils in a carrier oil found a big improvement in their symptoms over seven months, compared with just 15 per cent of those using carrier oils alone.[6]

❀ You might want to consider taking a flaxseed supplement to ensure you get your EFAs.

❀ Some hair supplements contain all the B vitamins, vitamin C, lysine and other nutrients you need for healthy hair growth.

❀ Some natural practitioners prescribe the mineral silicon to prevent hair loss. Horsetail is a good source of silicon.

❁ Use apple cider vinegar and sage tea as a rinse to help make hair shiny.

❁ Liquorice extract taken orally or used topically in a cream from a Traditional Chinese Medicine (TCM) practitioner may help prevent hair loss. As the kidneys reflect the quality of your hair, in TCM medicine taking supplements to support your kidneys (see Chapter 3) is considered important.

❁ Nettle tea may improve the quality of your hair. For extra shine, try rinsing your hair with nettle tea that has been strained and cooled. For dark hair, adding a teaspoon of vinegar or rosemary can add shine. The calming herb chamomile is traditionally used to lighten and brighten blonde hair.

❁ Raising your progesterone levels with natural progesterone cream can result in a fall in levels of androgen so that hair can grow back normally again. Talk to your doctor and never take without supervision as it is still technically a synthetically-produced medication. Be patient – hair growth is slow and it may take several months to notice a difference.

❁ Avoid hair products that are not natural, and avoid treating your hair roughly. Don't use a fine-toothed comb or towel-dry your hair. If you can, avoid using heated appliances on your hair; let it dry naturally.

The combination of optimum nutrition, stimulating scalp circulation (you might even like to try the odd headstand, or leaning forward with your head between your legs) and correcting hormonal imbalances has proved to be the most effective answer to hair loss. For more help, contact the alopecia associations listed in Chapter 12.

Hopefully this chapter will have given you useful information if specific PCOS symptoms are causing you special concern. Chapters 8 and 12 will give you more information and advice. Remember, if you do decide to visit an alternative or complementary therapist or take supplements you should tell your doctor you are doing so. A few doctors may still be resistant to the idea of natural therapies, but many doctors are starting to recognize that natural therapies are gathering more scientific and anecdotal evidence as well as helping patients feel more empowered and emotionally in control.

Adapting Your Diet for Your Health – When You Have PCOS and Diabetes, Thyroid Problems or Digestive Disorders

If you have diabetes, thyroid disease, or a digestive disorder such as IBS as well as PCOS, this chapter will look at how the right kind of diet can help.

PCOS AND DIABETES

Diabetes is thought to affect at least 16 million Americans and 2 million Britons. One survey suggests that one in five Britons has diabetes and that many are unaware of their condition. Diabetes is the third-leading cause of death after heart disease and cancer. The condition is becoming more common, with the number of those affected expected to double in the next 10 years.

Diabetes is generally divided into two categories. Type I diabetes is genetic or caused by pancreatic damage and requires insulin injection. Type II diabetes is more common than Type I diabetes. It is brought on by diet, lifestyle and genetic predisposition, which can show itself as PCOS insulin resistance.

Type I diabetes is caused by lack of insulin. As you know by now, insulin is responsible for the absorption of glucose into the liver, fat cells and muscles, which all need glucose for energy. If there is too little insulin, glucose levels in the blood rise. Symptoms of Type I diabetes include thirst, the need to urinate a lot, fatigue, hunger, weakness, weight loss and apathy.

The type of diabetes women with PCOS are at an increased risk of developing is Type II diabetes, also known as 'late onset' or 'age onset' diabetes. Women with PCOS who are overweight are most at risk of developing Type II diabetes (some experts believe that women with PCOS have a ninefold risk increase), as being overweight encourages insulin resistance. Women with Type II diabetes have plenty of insulin in their body, but their tissues become insensitive to it and don't use it well.

There is a grey area where insulin resistance stops and diabetes starts, and some experts would diagnose diabetes sooner than others, but if you feel tired most of the time, need to urinate a lot, are constantly thirsty and your vision is blurred, beyond a doubt you have diabetes and are not just PCOS insulin resistant.

Diabetes is a serious health risk and needs controlling because abnormally high levels of sugar in your blood can cause potentially serious problems. Diabetes of either type can contribute towards nerve damage, heart disease and arterial disease in the legs, high blood pressure, sight problems (including blindness) and kidney failure. If you have PCOS and any of the symptoms mentioned above, ask your doctor to carry out some blood and urine tests.

Blood-sugar levels can be corrected and controlled, and long-term health risks reduced, through medication and/or diet.

If you have diabetes your doctor will advise you on a diet to steady levels of blood glucose and help you lose or maintain a healthy weight (as excess weight makes diabetes worse). You may be given drugs to combat insulin resistance if you need them. It's important to understand that a sound diet for diabetes is about healthy eating and not just tailoring a regime that meets your needs in terms of blood glucose levels.

Completed in 1988, the Diabetes Control and Complications Trial (DCCT) 10-year National Institute of Health study of Americans with diabetes showed that eating a healthy, well-balanced diet results in better overall long-term health, fewer diabetic complications and an enhanced sense of physical and mental well-being. You'll also find that symptoms of PCOS improve.

When I was diagnosed with PCOS along with diabetes I felt that nobody could be so unlucky. But now that I've found a way of eating which can manage both conditions I feel a lot more positive and in control. I am living proof that with the right kind of diet and medication you don't have to endure a lifetime of poor health. Yes, sure I sometimes wish I didn't have to be quite so careful about my diet, but then I think about how good I feel and how much energy I've got and I stop feeling so sorry for myself.
Maria, 30

Dietary Strategies

The nutritional approach is fundamental if you have diabetes. Everything you eat and drink affects your blood-sugar levels and the way you feel.

Your daily diet won't be that different from the healthy PCOS diet. If you have PCOS and Type II diabetes, you pretty much need to eat the same as you would with PCOS anyway – and for women with PCOS who want to protect themselves from developing diabetes, the diet is also the same. However, while you can prevent or manage Type II diabetes with good eating and exercise, it is important to point out that if you have Type I you will always need your insulin injections alongside your healthy diet.

Your diet should consist of lots of water and about three regular meals and three regular snacks a day. It's important that you space your carbohydrates over the course of the day, and mix them with proteins and fats – for example eating dried beans and peas along with carbohydrate-rich foods to lower the effect of the carbohydrate-rich foods on your blood sugar. The glycemic index, which rates carbohydrates according to their effect on your blood sugar, should be used to determine which foods to avoid or which need to be combined with protein and fat. It's not as simple as avoiding sugary food and eating complex carbohydrates. You'll notice that table sugar does not raise blood-sugar levels as fast as some complex carbohydrates like white bread, and is no longer on the banned list from the British Diabetic Association.

Prevention Is Better than Cure

Cutting out sugar is not enough. You need to cut down on refined carbohydrates – because the body converts them into glucose too quickly. Eat foods with a low glycemic index which release their glucose slowly and steadily – wholemeal bread, pasta, rice and grains all fit the bill. Combine these with low-fat proteins such as tofu or beans and plenty of vegetables and fruit.

An ideal daily intake would be oat porridge, fruit and yogurt for breakfast, some nuts and fruit mid-morning, some low-fat protein and salad for lunch, a low-fat fruit smoothie mid-afternoon, and some low-fat protein, baked potato and vegetables for dinner. And keep your alcohol intake very low. We'd all do well to follow this diet for prevention, whether we have diabetes or not.

One important principle of a diet for diabetes is to eat foods which release sugar relatively slowly into the bloodstream, in the same ways as for PCOS. Conventional medical wisdom once held that starchy foods such as bread, potatoes, rice, pasta and cereals released sugar more slowly than sugary foods. However, during the past 20 years research has shown that starches often release sugar very quickly into the bloodstream. This is particularly true for potatoes and refined starches such as white bread, white rice and regular pasta. A study published in the *Journal of the American Medical Association* in 1997 found that women whose diets were rich in these foods had twice the risk of developing diabetes compared to women who eat a diet rich in wholegrains such as wholewheat pasta and wholemeal bread.[1]

It's important to understand, if you want to prevent Type II diabetes or have it already, that many starchy foods doctors and dieticians advise us to eat are simply bad for blood-sugar control and appear to increase the diabetes risk. A better diet is one based on moderate amounts of unrefined starch, along with other foods which release sugar relatively slowly into the bloodstream, including fresh fruits, beans and pulses. There is evidence that a diet rich in high fibre and low-GI complex carbohydrates can lower the risk of diabetes.

Health authorities are still arguing over the best levels of fats, proteins and carbohydrates in a diabetes diet, but it seems that the best anti-diabetes diet, according to most US and UK experts, is 50 to 60 per cent of your calories in healthy carbs such as wholegrains, pulses, fruits and vegetables, less than 30 per cent fats (less than 10 per cent saturated fats), and 30–40 grams of fibre a day.

Basically, a diet for diabetes, and the one recommended by both the British and American Diabetic Associations, is simply a healthy diet. It just needs to be fine-tuned. The majority of nutritional and lifestyle guidelines for people with diabetes are exactly the same as for any women looking after their present and future health and outlined in Chapter 2. There isn't any need to buy special diabetic foods.

Diabetes Strategies

To deal with the symptoms of diabetes which are distinct from those of PCOS, here is what you can do:

Your diet should be rich in high-fibre, slow sugar-releasing foods such as wholemeal and wholewheat pasta and fresh vegetables and fruit, with moderate amounts of lean protein and dairy produce. This reduces the need for insulin and also lowers the level of fats in your blood and the fibre helps to reduce blood-sugar swings.

Avoid: sugary, low-fibre foods, alcohol and transfatty acids (the latter are found in many processed foods, margarines, baked goods and fast foods). According to a recent study in the *American Journal of Clinical*

Medicine, it is not saturated fats but transfatty acids that are the problem, whereas polyunsaturated fats such as those found in oily fish (salmon, tuna, mackerel, herring) and many unrefined oils (sunflower, corn or flaxseed oil, for example) appear to reduce the risk of diabetes.[2]

Drink plenty of water throughout the day. This will help you excrete excess sugar from your body and also help the fibre in your diet perform its blood-regulatory functions.

Eat foods high in antioxidants, such as fresh fruits and vegetables, five times a day.

High-chromium foods such as grains and broccoli are useful because chromium helps control blood glucose levels. Other nutrients and foods that help normalize blood-sugar levels include spirulina, onions, cinnamon, fenugreek seeds, berries, brewer's yeast, cottage cheese, egg yolks, fish, garlic, kelp, soybeans and vegetables.

Get your protein from vegetable sources such as grains or legumes. Fish and low-fat dairy products are also acceptable sources of protein. Stick to foods that are low in animal fats and rich in high-fibre carbohydrates: beans, oats, wholegrains, nuts, fruits and vegetables.

Exercise provokes an insulin-like reaction in your body and is an important part of preventing and managing diabetes as well as PCOS. (We'll discuss exercise in more detail in Chapter 7.)

The largest study ever carried out on diabetes backs this up. Cutting back on calories from unhealthy, sugary and refined food sources and increasing physical activity can significantly reduce your risk. The US National Institutes of Health enrolled over 3,000 Americans who were at high risk because they were overweight, had relatives with diabetes, or had problems with processing blood sugar correctly, like many women with PCOS. Those that exercised moderately – say 30 minutes of walking five times a week – almost halved their risk of developing diabetes over the next few years.

Bill Hartnell of the charity Diabetes UK says that Type II diabetes is not the mild condition many of us may think. It can cause serious health problems, but 'the good news is that simple changes in lifestyle can make a dramatic difference and they are a very important part of prevention as well as managing the disease in those who have developed it'.

We'll discuss exercise in more detail in Chapter 7.

So, a wholesome, nutritious diet is the best way to boost your overall health if you have diabetes. The following dietary supplements also play their part:

Beta carotene	an important antioxidant, beta carotene is the non-toxic form of vitamin A, and is found in foods such as carrots, mangoes, oranges and sweet potatoes
B_3 (niacin)	found in fish, meat, nuts and wholegrains. Helps to control glucose levels
B_6 (pyridoxine)	found in cooked lentils and watermelon. Helps control glucose levels
Biotin	found in liver and egg yolk
Vitamin C	another important antioxidant – antioxidants are nutrients found in fruits and vegetables that are known to destroy or neutralize free radicals. Free radicals are naturally-occurring molecules in our bodies which contribute towards disease and ageing
Chromium	found in grains, broccoli, liver and pork. Early research suggests that chromium may also help you maintain healthy levels of HDL (the good cholesterol). Chromium polynicotinate is a nutritional supplement that can help control diabetes, but it is important that this supplement is taken under medical supervision as the effects on blood-sugar levels are very real and could result in a dangerous insulin reaction
Vitamin E	antioxidant
Magnesium	found in dairy products, nuts, vegetables and meat. Magnesium is also lacking in many women with PMS, so you could zap two birds with one stone
Selenium	antioxidant
Zinc	antioxidant

When choosing a multivitamin, look for one with plenty of B vitamins and antioxidants. If you take other supplements, check to see if you are already getting an adequate amount of certain vitamins or minerals in your multivitamin. (See Chapter 8 for more about these and other supplements.)

Supplementing with essential fatty acids may also be wise, as the science behind EFAs and health benefits proves that EFAs can positively affect many diseases, diabetes included.

Once you are eating a healthy diet – one that balances carbohydrates, proteins and fats and fills any nutrition gaps with supplements – you can look forward to improved blood-sugar control and optimum health, despite having diabetes and PCOS.

Natural Therapies

Having diabetes is stressful. It is an illness which demands constant attention and control. There are many gentle therapies which can soothe your mind and so enhance your control and management of the disease. Natural therapies don't promise to cure or prevent diabetes. What they can do, however, is help you feel more positive about yourself and encourage you to have a more positive approach to your health. They can also strengthen your body, relieve stress, improve glucose control and influence other diabetes- and PCOS-related symptoms.

The Power of Relaxation

Stress creates all sorts of imbalances in the body, so it becomes loaded with toxins. Stress-management is an important part of any diabetes self-help programme. Techniques such as tai chi and meditation will help reduce adrenaline and cortisol levels – both hormones which raise blood glucose levels – and consequently improve diabetes control.

Many people find simple techniques beneficial, including just sitting and *being* – sitting quietly and being aware of your breath flowing in and out.

'Transcendental mediation allows the body complete rest and a chance to let its own healing mechanisms work,' says TM teacher Jonathon Hinde.

High blood pressure can be a complication of diabetes. According to a study published in *Stroke*, the journal of the American Heart Association, just 20 minutes a day of transcendental meditation can help to control it.[3]

Among other therapies which have been found to be useful are aromatherapy, reflexology, autogenic training (a form of meditation which can help control blood-sugar levels and blood pressure) and counselling. Physical therapies which can reduce or alleviate some of the painful complications of diabetes, such as those affecting the nerves or circulation, are herbal remedies, acupuncture/acupressure, and yoga. Let's take a closer look at these techniques.

Herbal Medicine

A number of herbs can help stabilize blood-sugar levels. Two studies published in the *European Journal of Clinical Nutrition* reported that fenugreek improves glucose tolerance. Cinnamon may also be helpful, according to US researchers. Ginseng is currently under investigation as a treatment for diabetes. Research from Canada has shown that ginseng can reduce the rapid rise in blood-sugar levels when taken after a meal.[4]

Some herbs can have a rapid effect on blood-sugar levels, so it is important to consult your doctor or a qualified herbalist before trying herbal therapy. Herbs often used in the treatment of diabetes include: siberian ginseng, cedar berries, gymnema sylvestre, fenugreek, bitter lemon, garlic, juniper berries, cayenne pepper, huckleberry, buchu, dandelion root, uva ursi bilberry, ginkgo biloba and St John's Wort. St John's Wort is also helpful in relieving depression and anxiety. It is well known that emotional stress can have an impact on your blood-sugar levels.

A Chinese herbalist would treat diabetes with a combination of herbal remedies. Herbs used might include lilyturf root, grassy privet, lotus seed, Chinese yam and mulberry fruit, as well as dogwood fruit and water plaintain tuber. The herbalist may also suggest a soup of Chinese yam and Chinese wolfberry. Yam is rich in beta carotene, proteins and carbohydrates and strengthens the spleen, stomach, kidneys and lungs. Wolfberry seeds help restore the liver and kidneys, and are frequently used to treat diabetes.

According to Ayurvedic theory, diabetes is a metabolic *kapha*-type disorder caused by poor digestion which leads to high blood sugar. To control high blood sugar, an Ayurvedic practitioner might suggest treatments including a herbal supplement mixture, herbal massages or herbal steam baths. Several herbs – including bitter melon, neem and gymnema sylvestre – are believed to boost insulin production, increase sugar absorption by the cells and stimulate pancreatic activity.

Ayurvedic doctors also use turmeric as an effective treatment for controlling blood sugar. One way to take turmeric is to mix half a teaspoon of the spice with half a teaspoon of ground bay leaf mixed in 1 tablespoon of aloe vera juice. Take twice a day before lunch and dinner. When prescribed by a qualified practitioner, you can also simply add the spice to your cooking.

Since diabetes is viewed as a kapha-type disorder, an Ayurvedic practitioner might suggest following a kapha-pacifying diet: the avoidance of too many sweets, simple carbs and dairy products, and increasing your intake of fresh vegetables and bitter foods such as green bananas. Ayurvedic practitioners believe that protein can damage the kidneys, and fat can be difficult for those with diabetes to digest, so the amount of protein and fat in your diet will be closely monitored.

Warning: Because some herbs can have a rapid effect on blood-sugar levels and because this effect will vary from person to person, it's important to talk to your doctor before trying any herbal therapy. If you are on medication, some herbs may interact with your medication so your doctor should be involved.

Acupuncture

Acupuncture is the painless insertion of very fine disposable needles in points along the body's meridians to relieve symptoms by correcting energy imbalances and restoring the normal, healthy flow of energy. The World Health Organization endorses the use of acupuncture as a complementary treatment for diabetes. Acupuncture, in some studies, appears to be helpful for alleviating the pain suffered by those who have had diabetes over the long term. In terms of traditional Chinese medicine, diabetes is considered a stomach, kidney and spleen problem. Therefore the acupuncturist would target points along the meridians that correspond to these areas.

Acupressure uses many of the same points as acupuncturists, but the practitioner uses deep finger pressure instead of needles. The technique is believed to stimulate the circulatory and endocrine system and can be particularly helpful for stress-related symptoms such as headaches, anxiety and insomnia as well as digestive problems, muscle aches and menstrual problems.

Yoga

The practice of yoga (part of the Ayurvedic system of healthcare) is designed to quiet the mind by teaching you how to pay attention to your breathing and to the movement or stillness of your body through a series of postures. Yoga is very popular right now, especially among those who are seeking gentler forms of exercise after years of bone-jarring aerobics and jogging. Combined with walking and/or swimming, yoga can help you get all the exercise you need for flexibility, heart health and strong bones.

According to a study published in *Diabetes Research and Clinical Practice*, yoga has been proved beneficial for people with diabetes. If you have diabetes, yoga can stimulate feelings of calm and tranquillity and enhance your feelings of control. It may also help reduce blood glucose levels, lower blood pressure and control weight. Many people find the gentle movements and relaxing breathing exercises of yoga beneficial when it comes to pain and stiffness, and relieving fatigue.

Yoga therapy is when a teacher creates a tailor-made yoga programme for you specially to help with your particular health problems. To find your nearest practitioner, see Chapter 12.

PCOS AND THYROID PROBLEMS

I was diagnosed with PCOS in my teens, then in my late twenties I seemed to lose all my energy and the pounds piled on. Very quickly I turned from a woman who would go to aerobics twice a week, play with my two children and go to sleep at around midnight to someone who could barely get out of bed. My weight soared by nearly 30 pounds and I was constantly trying to hide my body. Emotionally I was a wreck. I suffered mood swings and I lost my temper easily. I'd lash out at my boyfriend and even shout at the kids over stupid things. When my periods stopped completely I went to see the doctor. I was diagnosed with hypothyroidism.
Dawn, 27

One in 10 adults is thought to have thyroid problems, so it's not surprising to find that one in 10 women with PCOS has them, too. If you feel irritable, nervous and hot a lot of the time and suffer from any of the following – irritable bowel, fatigue, insomnia, hair loss, weight loss, irregular periods and sometimes goitres and protruding eyeballs – you could have *hyperthyroidism* (an overactive thyroid). Hyperthyroidism occurs when the thyroid gland produces too much thyroid hormone, resulting in an overactive metabolism.

Hypothyroidism (underactive thyroid) is even more common. Here, the thyroid gland produces too little thyroid hormone. Symptoms of an underactive thyroid include fatigue, weight gain, irregular periods, dry skin, depression, poor concentration and intolerance to cold. If you constantly feel cold while others around you are hot, you may be suffering from reduced thyroid function.

Thyroid problems are more common among men than women. They can cause many illnesses, and may in women trigger symptoms of PCOS. Alternatively, PCOS can trigger the symptoms of thyroid problems. This is because the pituitary gland, thyroid gland and sex glands all work together and are influenced by thyroid function. If there is a problem in one gland, they may all be affected. And don't forget that PCOS, like a thyroid disorder, challenges your body's normal metabolism.

Because the symptoms of thyroid disorder can often be confused with those of PCOS and vice versa, it is important that you see your doctor to determine if you have PCOS, a thyroid disorder, or both.

Dietary Strategies: Overactive Thyroid (Hyperthyroidism)

Eat plenty of the following foods: broccoli, Brussels sprouts, cabbage, cauliflower, kale, mustard greens, peaches, pears, soybeans, spinach and turnips. Many nutritionists believe that these foods contain nutrients which can help to suppress thyroid hormone production. Avoid dairy products and stimulants such as coffee, tea, nicotine and soft drinks.

Because digestion speeds up with this disorder, malabsorption often occurs, so a healthy, balanced diet is essential.

Supplements include a good multivitamin and mineral complex. Increased amounts of vitamins and minerals are needed for this hyper-metabolic condition. Ensure that your multivitamin contains vitamin C, E and B complex, especially B_1, B_2 and B_6, needed for normal thyroid function. Brewer's yeast, essential fatty acids and lecithin granules may also be helpful.

Dietary Strategies: Underactive Thyroid (Hypothyroidism)

According to naturopathic consultant Martin Budd, who treats people with thyroid problems, symptoms of hypothyroidism can be greatly alleviated through diet and weight loss. He recommends a low-fat and low-sugar diet which uses the glycemic index (see page 27) to make the correct food choices.

The term 'Mediterranean Triad' was first coined by Paul Kendrick to describe the three key elements of the regional diets of Greece, Italy and southern France – places where the incidence of diabetes and hypothyroidism is low. The aim of the diet is to eat whole-grain products and fresh fruits and vegetables, and to reduce the intake of total fat and sugar by substituting olive oil and other oils for solid fats and replacing fatty red meat with lean meat. Once again we are looking at a basic healthy diet, as described in Chapter 2.

Iodine deficiency is associated with thyroid problems and goitres. If the following foods, which reduce iodine function, form a major part of your diet and you are suffering from thyroid deficiency, you need to limit your intake: Brussels sprouts, peaches, pears, spinach, turnips, cruciferous plants such as cabbage, cauliflower, sprouts, soya, broccoli, kale and mustard greens, maize, sweet corn, millet, peanuts, almonds, walnuts, and mustard and rape seeds.
Avoid processed and refined foods, including white sugar and flour, which can trigger swings in blood sugar.
Avoid fluoride (including that found in toothpaste and tap water) and chlorine (also found in tap water). Chlorine and fluoride can block receptors in the thyroid gland, resulting in reduced thyroid function.
Helpful supplements include kelp, vitamin B complex, essential fatty acids, iron, vitamins A, C and E and the minerals selenium, manganese, copper, iron and zinc.

Natural Therapies

Like PCOS, all thyroid symptoms have an impact on your mind as well as your body. So therapies that act on your body via the mind and vice versa are likely to be particularly helpful. For instance, meditation and yoga can help to calm a racing mind. Tai chi and yoga may help to raise your energy levels and mood. Aromatherapy is likely to be helpful, too, as the essential oils work gently on your mind and body to rebalance mind and mood. Rosemary, for example, can relax away tension, basil lifts your mood, lavender is relaxing and lemon balm can help you sleep peacefully.

A medical herbalist might recommend the herbs bayberry, black cohosh and golden seal in a tailor-made prescription to help an underactive thyroid.

An ancient Ayurvedic herbal remedy using the extract of the guggulu tree has proven effective in normalizing cholesterol levels and stimulating the thyroid.

My hypothyroidism meant that my metabolism was working slowly, which was why I was getting heavier and didn't have any energy. To be honest at that point I was just pleased to find out why I'd been feeling so ill. I started to think I was going crazy. Thyroxine tablets were prescribed for my thyroid and an exercise plan along with a daily multivitamin and mineral supplement. I also read some slimming magazines and started to cut down my portion sizes. Within weeks I felt better. I lost weight and my periods returned. I was able to attend my weekly exercise classes again.

Although my body isn't back to normal yet, it's getting there. Most important, my confidence has returned and I feel like my old self again.
Dawn, 27

Finding the right natural therapy is a matter of personal taste, but the following may be particularly suited to the treatment of thyroid problems. If you do use natural therapies, it must always be in consultation with your doctor.

Acupuncture

According to the tenets of traditional Chinese medicine, disease occurs when the body's internal balance is disrupted in some way. Harmony and balance depend on the smooth flow of the body's life-force, or *chi*, which circulates along invisible pathways or channels. This smooth flow also depends on the correct balance of two qualities called *yin* (feminine) and *yang* (masculine). Shortage of yin manifests in symptoms of coldness, fatigue, depression – all the symptoms of an underactive thyroid. A shortage of yang would manifest in the symptoms of an overactive thyroid.

An acupuncturist would aim to restore your body's natural balance of yin and yang, and strengthen the chi.

Autogenic Training

Autogenic training is one of the few alternative therapies that has been studied in relation to thyroid problems. Autogenic training involves a series of exercises designed to focus your mind on feelings of heaviness, warmth in the limbs, a calm heartbeat, easy natural breathing, abdominal warmth and cooling of the forehead. You repeat the exercises three times a day after meals for about 10 minutes. The therapy draws on the insights of meditation and is particularly useful for mild anxiety states. The techniques have been found to lower heart rate and blood pressure, and improve emotional balance. As far as specific thyroid symptoms are concerned, research has shown that a number of typical symptoms of an overactive thyroid, such as sweating, irritability and nausea, diminish over the course of autogenic training.

PCOS AND DIGESTIVE DISORDERS

Some days food goes straight through me. I have to make sure I am near a restroom. My stomach always seems to be churning and it makes me feel tired and irritable. I'm sure I'm not getting my nutrients and that isn't helping my hair loss.
Hannah, 37

Many women with PCOS have digestive problems, especially constipation and IBS (irritable bowel syndrome). Research is being undertaken to see why IBS is often linked with PCOS, but it may have something to do with the slightly lowered metabolic rate after a meal that is common among women with PCOS. Food takes longer to digest, or isn't digested efficiently, and this can lead to digestive problems such as IBS, constipation, or bouts of diarrhoea.

Food Combining

If you have digestive problems, a food-combining diet may be able to help.

Food-combining diets draw their inspiration from the work of Dr William Howard Hay, who recommended that we cut down on protein, starches and highly processed foods, increase our intake of vegetables, fruits and salads and don't mix foods that fight. The final suggestion – don't mix foods that fight – is the trademark of food-combining diets. Eating several different food types at one meal is a modern habit and, according to Dr Hay, not necessarily a healthy one.

To understand the food-combining theory you need to think about the typical mixed meal many of us have. Starch (perhaps potatoes, rice, bread, pasta or grains) is mixed with a protein (meat, fish, eggs, cheese, milk) with possibly a vegetable or two or a fruit. Given that proteins take longer to digest than starches, and starches take longer than vegetables or fruits, mixing them all up together can cause digestive confusion.

Although it is the opposite theory to combining protein and carbs to maintain steady blood-sugar levels in PCOS, if you have digestive problems the benefits of food combining can mean you get more nutrients. You can use it to see if it helps settle your problems down and then start trying to mix proteins and carbs again, or you may find it suits you just fine to food combine. Every woman with PCOS is different, so it's up to us to experiment and find what works for us.

Putting the Food Combining Rules into Practice

1 Don't mix starch foods or sugars with proteins.
2 Increase your intake of alkaline-forming, nutrient-rich fresh vegetables, fruits and salads.
3 Keep all fruits away from main meals.
4 Don't mix milk with protein or starch.
5 Avoid processed, refined foods.

Try to base your diet on 20 per cent acid-forming foods and 80 per cent alkali-forming foods. Acid-forming foods include all kinds of meat and fish, cheese, eggs, all grains except millet, all kinds of bread, flour and sugar, peas, beans, legumes and nuts. Wholegrain products are less acid-forming than white rice or flour. Pickles and sauces are all acid-forming, as are tea, coffee and alcohol. Milk, yogurt, butter and vegetable oils are regarded as neutral foods. Most fruits and vegetables, as well as millet, are alkaline-forming.

Not only will these changes help you avoid mixing foods that fight, so that your digestive system improves, but they will also improve the quality of your diet. Everyone should increase the amount of fresh fruits and vegetables they eat and steer clear of processed, refined foods which have a detrimental effect on the efficacy of your digestion, your symptoms and your health.

Meal Times

The best time for the important alkaline meal is breakfast. Try fresh fruit, or fruit with plain yogurt and a tablespoon of wheatgerm plus a hot drink such as weak tea, herbal tea or coffee.

The best time for carbohydrates is at midday: a salad with jacket potatoes served with butter and steamed vegetables, a sweet fruit such as a banana to follow. For a packed lunch: a salad sandwich with wholemeal bread and butter, a thermos of vegetable soup and a compatible fruit make a satisfying meal. Fruits compatible with starch meals include bananas, raisins, dates, figs, grapes, pears, currants and sultanas.

The evening meal is the time for protein: raw vegetables and or vegetable soup with a portion of fish, meat, chicken, game, eggs or cheese and lightly steamed green or root vegetables followed by a compatible fruit. Fruits compatible with protein meals include apples, apricots, berries, grapefruit, lemons, oranges, peaches, pears, pineapples, strawberries and tangerines.

Maintaining a healthy weight is an essential part of a healthy lifestyle, but it can be a problem area if you have PCOS. In the next chapter we'll discuss what you can do on top of your basic diet to help you lose weight.

Losing Weight – Breaking the PCOS Cycle

'I only have to look at food and I put on weight' is the classic line many women with PCOS use to describe their relationship to food.

My doctor told me that a lot of my PCOS symptoms would get better if I lost some weight. But the truth is I eat like a bird. OK, I have the odd glass of wine here and there, but on the whole I don't eat much more than anyone else. I'm beginning to think that I am just meant to be overweight.
Ruth, 35

You know that saying 'A minute on your lips, a lifetime on your hips'? It must have been written with me in mind. I've tried every diet you can think of, but I never lose more than a couple of pounds. Losing weight is hard. Trying to lose weight when you are diagnosed with PCOS feels like cycling up a steep hill with the wind pushing you back time and time again.
Louise, 28

I have been trying to diet for months. I watched my best friend successfully whittle down to her goal, but I'm totally stuck. I've joined a gym and I do manage to make very slow headway, but it is a ton of work and perseverance and I bounce back up on the scales with the snap of my fingers. I started to lose my hair first. Then came the weight gain. I think for many of us, the weight gain is our biggest challenge. There doesn't seem to be a pat answer. If anyone can condense all this into something simple, it would be such a relief. How do I win the battle?
Susannah, 43

If you have weight to lose, success can not only make you look and feel better but can also be a very effective way to treat your symptoms. Studies of women with PCOS who are overweight have shown that excess weight can make the symptoms worse, and that weight loss sees an improvement.[1] But if you have PCOS you may find losing weight frustrating and difficult.

THE PCOS WEIGHT TRAP

According to research, the rate at which food is broken down after a meal and used by your body (*postprandial thermogenesis*) is reduced in women with PCOS.[2] 'This can predispose women with polycystic ovary syndrome to weight gain,' says Dr Helen Mason, senior lecturer in Reproductive Technology at St George's Hospital Medical School, London. Postprandial thermogenesis actually accounts for around 80 per cent of the calories burned by your body over the course of a day. According to Dr Robert Franklin, Clinical Professor of Obstetrics and Gynecology at Baylor College of Medicine in Houston, Texas, it is also thought that higher-than-average levels of testosterone, which all women with PCOS have, are linked with a tendency to hold on to body fat.

Add to this the insulin resistance problem – which blocks the action of hormones that can help you burn off fat for energy, and also traps you in a cycle of blood-sugar ups and downs – and you are in the PCOS weight trap. You crave foods that give you a blood-sugar rush, but store them so well that you put on weight, without being able to shift it. In other words, a woman with PCOS eating the same seven days' worth of food as a woman without may store as many calories as if she had eaten eight days' worth!

Means of Escape

So what can you do if you want or need to lose weight?

It won't surprise you to learn that the first essential step is to eat a healthy, balanced diet like that outlined in Chapter 2, which will help stabilize your blood-sugar levels, reduce any food cravings and set you on the right path. The next step is to start adding things on top of your basic diet to help you lose weight: cutting down your portion sizes, fighting carb cravings and hunger pangs, taking food supplements, getting motivated and starting up a regular exercise routine. We'll also take a look at fluid-retention and the contraceptive pill, either of which could be adding to your inability to lose weight effectively.

PORTION CONTROL

Hormones, toxins and PCOS can affect the rate at which you burn calories, but the basic formula for weight loss remains the same: 'We try to explain to our clients the importance of energy balance,' say Sally Wharmby and Claire Mellors, senior dietitians from Queens Medical Centre, Nottingham, who run weight-loss clinics for women with PCOS. 'Eating more food than you need will lead to weight gain, but this is something you can control by the food and exercise choices you make.'

The easiest way to gradually reduce your food intake without skimping on the nutrients you need to burn fat is to cut down on your portion size. Every meal should still be a balance of carbs, proteins and fats.

If you follow the guidelines in Chapter 2 you should be getting a balanced diet with sufficient vitamins and minerals. Just watch your serving size. As a rough guide, according to the US Department of Agriculture, you need:

2–3 servings of meat, fish, eggs, beans and nuts a day	1 serving = one egg, half a cup of beans, or meat or fish about the size of a clenched fist
2–3 servings of milk, yogurt or cheese a day (or of non-dairy produce, like soya or nut milk, if you are intolerant)	1 serving = about 2 oz of cheese or 1 cup of milk or yogurt

4–6 servings of whole grains a day	1 serving = 1 slice of bread, a bowl of cereal, or half a cup of rice or pasta
4 servings of fruit	1 serving = 1 piece of fruit
5 servings of vegetables	1 serving = half a cup of raw or cooked vegetables
Fats and oils	in moderation

Sample Daily Menu

Breakfast
Bowl of oatbran cereal with skimmed milk
1 boiled egg
2 slices of whole wheat bread with low fat spread

Snack
Apple with a handful of nuts

Lunch
Low-fat cottage cheese salad with tomatoes, red onions, boiled rice, fresh herbs and sweetcorn
Fruit salad

Snack
Low-fat yogurt with dried fruits and sesame seed crackers

Dinner
Steamed fish with new potatoes and a variety of vegetables
1 peach poached in white wine

Portion sizes have got bigger and bigger over the years. As a result, waistlines have got bigger too. Proper attention paid to serving size will encourage the slow, gradual weight loss you should aim for. Start checking your servings now, and make a few small reductions. You don't need to cut out your favourite dishes – just don't eat too much of them.

If you are concerned that smaller portion sizes won't satisfy your hunger, there are lots of things you can do to help you get that full feeling.

I've found it really helpful to divide up the food on my plate. As long as half of it is vegetables, a quarter protein and the rest carbs, I know I am doing OK. PCOS can make dieting seem very complicated, but this simple strategy has worked wonders for me. I've lost 10 pounds in six months.
Lucinda, 33

✿ Take time over your meals. Put down your knife and fork after each mouthful and chew your food slowly.
✿ If you think you want a second helping or dessert, wait 10 of 15 minutes and see if you are still hungry.
✿ Don't shop or cook when you are really hungry. Make sure that you never let yourself get that hungry by keeping a supply of healthy, low-fat snacks nearby.
✿ Remember that it will take time to adjust to smaller portion sizes. Your stomach may have stretched after a long period of overeating so that it needs more food to help you feel full.
✿ If you are overeating for emotional reasons, see the advice in Chapter 11.

Weight-loss Diet Tips

Avoiding large snacks and changing your routine to smaller, more frequent snacks will help satisfy your appetite and regulate cravings. Around six small meals a day is helpful if you want to lose weight. Most nutritionists agree that eating little and often is the most effective way to promote weight loss. You should also stop eating several hours before you go to bed, say 8 p.m. This is because when you go to bed your body needs to rest, not digest. It doesn't make sense to eat a lot of food when all you are going to do is sleep. The earlier in the day you eat, the more likely you are to burn off calories even if you are sitting down a lot.

Below are some other tips, tricks and strategies from women with PCOS that you might find helpful:

Chocolate and white bread have always been my downfall. I know they were making me feel worse and causing my acne to flare up, but I can't live without them. My dietician told me to get rid of them, but this was too radical. What's working better for me is to include them in my diet once in a while so I don't feel deprived.
Amelia, 39

Drinking a couple of glasses of water 20 minutes before a meal always helps me. I find that I'm not so hungry and less tempted to eat foods which I know will make me gain weight and my acne worse.
Becky, 19

When I stopped eating fatty, sugary snacks and ate vegetables or fruit instead, the pounds melted away and my periods came bang on schedule.
Marion, 29

It was incredible – as soon as I started eating breakfast and having lighter lunches and suppers I started to lose weight and my periods came back. I don't eat anything after 7 p.m. now. I'm sleeping better and I wake up in the morning feeling slim and energetic.
Sheila, 41

Eating out was my downfall. I work in advertising and a lot of the time have to take clients out to dinner. But I've learned that eating out doesn't have to be a nightmare if I follow the same rules I do at home: avoid pastry, deep fried foods, mayonnaise, oily dressings and cream or cheese sauces. I always ask for dressings to be served on the side, and look for grilled, poached, stir-fried or steamed dishes. I eat slowly and steer clear of the dessert trolley.
Clara, 34

To Count or not to Count?

There are two schools of thought on counting calories. One believes that calorie-counting is detrimental and takes the focus away from nutrients if you are trying to lose weight. The other believes that calorie-counting is the only effective way to lose weight, because if you take in more calories than you use, you will gain weight. You have to find what works best for you. If you do decide to count calories, make sure you get your calorie needs assessed by a doctor, dietician or nutritionist and that you don't miss out on nutrients in an effort to reduce your calorie count. Remember – one packet of biscuits could give you a day's calories, but it won't keep you healthy!

Nutrient-rich Foods that Can Help You Lose Weight

The more nutrient-rich foods you eat, the slimmer you'll get – and you won't feel hungry all the time, either. Vegetables are the ultimate diet miracle food. They are filling but low in calories. Here are a few examples of nutrient-rich foods which can actually help you lose weight:

Wholegrain bread	This has chromium, the metabolism-boosting mineral that helps you shed stored fat. It also contains iron, which plays an important part in the burning of energy from the food you eat.
Wholewheat bread	Contains niacin, which helps release energy from the food you eat.
Bananas	Contain potassium. Potassium flushes sodium out of the body and can help you lose weight. Women who have more potassium in their diet burn calories faster than those who don't. (Cantaloupe is another good food source of potassium.) Bananas also contain magnesium, indispensable for weight loss. It is involved in every major biological process in the body. Bananas do have a high GI, though, so make sure you eat them with a handful of nuts to stabilize blood-sugar levels.
Broccoli	Your body burns calories simply by chewing broccoli. Broccoli also contains vitamins B_2 and B_6, essential for carbohydrate and fat metabolism and the breakdown of protein.

Black-eyed peas	High in zinc. Zinc is an important nutrient for weight loss. It is also associated with the proper functioning of insulin.
Spinach	Contains iodine, which helps the body metabolize excess fat.
Lean meats	The protein in lean meat such as chicken helps you convert fat into muscle. Muscle burns more calories than fat. Protein also takes longer to digest than carbohydrate, so eating it keeps you satisfied longer and prevents snacking.
Fibre-rich foods	Kidney beans, fibre-rich vegetables and bran cereals expand in our stomachs, filling us up with fewer calories. Adequate fibre ensures healthy digestion. It can block the absorption of fat, too.
Eggs	Rich in biotin, needed for the release of energy from carbohydrates, for fat-burning and for the breakdown of amino acids. (Other food sources of biotin include legumes, milk, cereal and nuts.) Eggs also contain vitamin B_5 (important for energy and tissue metabolism) and phosphorus (needed for the normal function of many of the B vitamins involved in energy production). The whites of eggs are protein sources which contain the amino acid L-carnitine which studies have shown unlocks the fat stored in our cells and enables it to be burned for energy.
Strawberries	Like all fruits, strawberries are high in vitamin C. Vitamin C is essential for weight loss because it is involved in the metabolism of amino acids.
Wholewheat pasta	This boosts serotonin levels. Serotonin is the 'feel-good' hormone that can stop food cravings.
Green leafy vegetables	These are high in vitamin E. Vitamin E protects your body from toxins when you lose weight.

CARBOHYDRATE CRAVINGS

If I pass a cake shop or smell fresh bread baking I find it impossible to resist. I have to buy some. It's the same at home. If there are biscuits in the tin I can't resist them. Sometimes my cravings for potato and rice are so strong people think I must be pregnant. Luckily I don't have a weight problem, but I do feel tired a lot and get horrible outbursts of acne.
Melissa, 24

Many women with PCOS find they are fighting carbohydrate cravings. This is probably because starchy foods – from doughnuts and biscuits to white bread, rice and potatoes – send your blood sugar rocketing very quickly after you eat them. But with such high levels of circulating blood sugar your body screams for insulin in order to be able to store the sugar away and out of your bloodstream where it can do harm. But when you are insulin resistant your body needs to pump out an awful lot of insulin before the tissues respond and start storing that blood sugar away. This means that the levels of insulin are so high that your body stores nearly all your blood sugar away and you go from one extreme to the other. The resulting dip in blood sugar means you feel tired and sleepy, craving the high glucose foods all over again and staying trapped in the carbohydrate craving cycle.

If you choose the healthy fresh foods we have talked about in Chapter 2 and then use the GI Index to refine your choice even more, you can really help yourself. For instance, you know you need to eat more fruits, and if you use the GI Index to choose low GI-fruits you can help yourself even more.

One problem with making hard-and-fast rules according to the GI, which gives GI rankings based on the effect of a single food eaten on its own, is that the GI of a given food depends not only on the type of carbohydrate you have eaten but on how much is eaten, what other foods are eaten at the same time and how the food is cooked. Another problem is that different women have different reactions to the same foods. You are an individual with PCOS, and that means you must determine how particular foods affect your blood-sugar levels and the way you look and feel. Once again we return to the theme of a balanced diet. It's not only about choosing the right carbohydrates, it's about balancing those carbohydrates and making sure you eat them with the right proteins and fats.

You don't have to ban foods containing a high glycemic index from your diet. However, you can use the information to plan meals that help control your blood-sugar levels. Legumes, for instance, have a low glycemic index, and when you eat them along with other carbohydrate-rich foods they can actually lower the glycemic effect of those other foods on your blood sugar. Nuts, bran and dried fruits can do the same. So try sprinkling some chopped nuts on your breakfast cereal, or eating legumes such as chickpeas with a rice dish.

The glycemic index is not meant to be interpreted as a list of good or bad foods, but is simply a guide to better food choices. Fixing yourself a sandwich? White and French breads have a high glycemic index; rye and sourdough breads are moderate on the scale.

Food Craving	Low-GI Alternative
Processed biscuits/crackers made with refined white flour	Products containing whole grains and or dried fruits
White or brown rice	Brown basmati rice or parboiled rice
Cakes and muffins made with refined white flour	Products containing whole grains and or dried fruits
Potatoes	Legumes (lentil, soybeans, baked beans) or wholegrain pasta
Bananas, tropical fruits	Apples, oranges, peaches and plums
Ice cream	Skimmed milk and frozen yogurt
Jelly Beans	Chocolate

Sugar-busting Tips

Don't go shopping when you are hungry – you'll end up buying sugary foods.

Stock up on healthier snacks (see list on page 52).

Get some hot chocolate and make a cup with skimmed milk or soya milk.

Explore your health food store. Rice cakes with banana and pure fruit spread or peanut butter make delicious snacks.

For a comfort fix, make yourself a bowl of oatmeal porridge with honey.

Keep fresh fruit, dried fruit and healthy snacks such as vegetable sticks nearby so you don't give in to the temptation to get yourself an unhealthy snack.

Smelling vanilla essence oil can help prevent cravings for sweet foods, according to research from St George's Hospital, London.[3] Dab a couple of drops on a tissue and inhale when you feel the need.

I was diagnosed with PCOS when I was 18. My doctor put me on the Pill to regularize my periods. It was then that the weight started piling on, not just a couple of pounds, but a stone and then another and another. I had slight blonde facial hair, which had grown down the side of my face to make sideburns. It was very noticeable. My periods stopped and I felt awful. I was unhappy with the Pill, so the doctor changed it, which made me much worse.

I tried to keep positive and keep my chin up – or should I say 'chins' in my case?! Soon I was shaving my face nearly every day. In early 2001 I hit rock bottom and got very depressed.

Things began to change for the better when I moved and my new doctor referred me to a dietician with experience in designing diets for women with PCOS. To my complete surprise I lost 13 pounds in 2 weeks. Like most women with PCOS, I have joined countless slimming organizations and got bored on week 2, as I always lost a lot of weight week 1 but then nothing, so I wasn't really hoping for much. The dietician explained that I wasn't losing weight because my metabolism was slow and the fact that I was taking medication (I'm on metformin). It was an eye opener, the first person in years who wasn't blaming me for being overweight. She personalized a PCOS diet for me, based on my slow metabolism and blood-sugar problems.

To date I have lost a big 20 pounds in 4 weeks. I am thrilled. I am never hungry because I have to eat every few hours to help my metabolic rate to speed up, and the weight is still falling off! My acne is clearing and I've got masses of energy. I'm also taking lots of supplements to help my PCOS. I take a multivitamin and mineral supplement, flax seed for Omega-3, vitex (chaste tree berry) to help balance my hormones, and milk thistle and nettle tincture to help my liver process and eliminate toxins. I also use saw palmetto to help with the excess facial hair growth (and yes, ladies, I can see a definite improvement with this!).

I feel a different woman to the woman I was a year ago. I think I'm living proof that PCOS doesn't have to mean a lifetime problem with your weight and your self-esteem. You don't have to feel helpless. Whether or not you take medication (I'm still on metformin) there are lots of things you can do to help yourself.

Stephanie, 30

CONSTANT HUNGER

I was constantly hungry. I was hungry from the minute I got up to the minute I went to bed. I felt like a slave to food. I blamed PCOS, but it wasn't PCOS that was causing the problem – it was the food I was eating and the way I was eating it. I wasn't eating protein or fat with my carbohydrate, so my stomach never felt full.

Maeve, 19

If you constantly feel hungry, a diet of protein, fats and carbs at every meal may help you. The theory is that because excess insulin makes you crave food all the time, eating fewer carbohydrates and including more fat and protein in your diet become important tools for reducing insulin, food cravings and weight gain. Since the foundation stone of the Zone diet is lowering insulin levels, it can be particularly helpful if you have blood-sugar problems and feel hungry all the time.

According to Dr Barry Sears, creator of the Zone diet (which has proved useful for many women with PCOS), if we control the amount of protein we eat we can control our health and well-being. He also believes that food isn't just fuel for the human machine. It also controls hormone levels. The Zone diet claims to help fight heart disease, diabetes, fatigue and depression and keep all the hormonal systems working smoothly.

On the Zone diet you need to ensure that every meal you eat has a good balance of carbohydrate, fat and protein. Eating 40 per cent complex carbohydrates, 30 per cent protein and 30 per cent fat can moderate insulin levels and keep you feeling fuller for longer.

Zone Rules

The Zone diet is not a low-carb or high-protein diet. Dr Sears stresses you should never eat more protein than you can fit in the palm of your hand at any meal – and that this should be balanced by at least an equal-sized portion of healthy carbs such as vegetables or brown rice. He also stresses a moderate amount of fat in sauces and spreads is a good idea, and insists you don't let more than a few hours go between meals.

The basics of the Zone diet can provide a useful plan for you to follow in order to fulfil the 10-step healthy diet from Chapter 2. Just make sure that the fats you take in are high in Omega-3 wherever possible, and don't cut out healthy carbohydrates.

Also remember, exercise is a vital part of any PCOS diet plan because it lowers insulin resistance – the Zone plan also stresses this.

Little and Often

Eating little and often can help you if you feel hungry all the time. If there is a long gap between meals, your blood glucose will drop to a low level, leaving you tired and lacking in energy. Because of your brain's absolute requirement for glucose you start to break down muscle to provide the glucose. The net effect is a loss in muscle mass, reduction in metabolic rate, fatigue, lack of concentration and swings in blood sugar.

Give your body food every few hours to boost your metabolic rate and keep your blood-sugar levels stable. Develop a grazing mentality and eat little and often. And don't forget to balance carbohydrate snacks with a little piece of protein to prevent rapid swings in blood sugar:

- ❀ salad sandwich with nuts or a dollop of hummus
- ❀ rice cake with chopped banana or pure fruit spread
- ❀ teacakes with low-fat cream cheese
- ❀ 1 tablespoon natural peanut butter on celery
- ❀ One low-fat yogurt with a rye cracker
- ❀ $^1/_3$ cup low-fat cottage cheese with bread sticks
- ❀ $^1/_4$ cup low-fat cottage cheese and half a piece of fruit
- ❀ 1 cup vegetable soup with seeds and bread roll.

Low-carbohydrate Diets: Good for PCOS?

Many low-carbohydrate diets are being touted as cures for PCOS weight gain. The logic is: if the root of PCOS is an inability to respond properly to insulin, many symptoms can be cured or even eliminated by restricting foods which produce too much insulin. Since your body produces insulin every time you eat carbohydrates, the best thing to do is to restrict the consumption of carbohydrates.

But is cutting down or cutting out carbs good for your health?

First of all, any diet that recommends cutting out carbs altogether or restricting them severely should be avoided. Carbohydrates are an essential source of energy, vitamins, minerals and fibre. If you cut carbs drastically or altogether, your brain and body will lack the energy they need to function optimally. Metabolism will slow, so you will put on weight on less food. You will feel tired and lethargic and find it hard to concentrate.

With PCOS you need to cut out refined carbs and choose instead the *right*, low-GI carbs such as vegetables and pulses.

Rapid weight loss based on eating low-carbohydrate, high-protein foods pose potential health threats and may be ineffective in the long term. A study by the American Heart Association found that very low-carbohydrate diets are missing vital vitamins and minerals and tend to be high in fat, increasing the risk of heart disease.[4] A report in the Association's journal, *Circulation*, has also raised questions about the health benefits of such regimes.[5] Any diet that puts too much emphasis on high protein isn't good for your health. Lots of protein puts pressure on the kidneys, which have to filter out the harmful toxins produced by the extra intake. Plus it's a dreadful diet if you are vegetarian. Pushing up protein intake can also increase the loss of calcium in the body, which can lead to osteoporosis. Too much fat can lead to weight gain and poor health. In addition, you could feel too weak from lack of carbohydrates to exercise, and you won't be getting the fibre and nutrients your body needs. Finally, a very low-carb diet is very boring and hard to sustain in the long term.

As long as carbohydrate intake isn't restricted to less than 40 per cent of your food, however, lower-carbohydrate diets can be helpful. If you want to balance your blood-sugar levels, lose weight and minimize your risk of insulin resistance, you shouldn't be cutting down on carbs, you should be eating the right kinds of complex, low-GI carbs as part of a balanced diet packed with fresh fruit and veg, high-quality protein, wholegrains and EFAs.

Ketosis – Medical No-carb Dieting

Ketosis is a weight-reduction method used by some US dieticians for people with real weight problems. The idea is to make someone lose weight as rapidly as occurs in starvation, but to give enough protein and supplements to prevent the body injuring itself. The most well known is the Protein-Sparing Modified Fast (PSMF) developed by Professor George Blackburn at the Massachusetts Institute of Technology. This employs a few hundred calories of high-protein food, supplements for vitamins and minerals, and no carbohydrates whatsoever. The PSMF produces an altered biological state in which fat is broken down very rapidly. This state is called ketosis because fat breakdown products known as ketone bodies accumulate in the blood and can be measured in the urine. After a few days appetite is suppressed and a sense of energy and well-being ensues.

This diet has its limitations. The first is that it is very hard to stick to. The second is that if you go off the diet and eat carbohydrate, this can cause rapid and dangerous swings in blood sugar. The third is that it must be overseen by a doctor. The PSMF is serious medicine – it must not and cannot be carried out on your own with any degree of safety.

EXERCISE

Exercise, in combination with a healthy diet, is an essential weight-loss tool for anyone who wants to lose weight. For women with PCOS, it is particularly beneficial. Not only can it kick-start weight loss but it has been proven to help achieve proper insulin levels, which in turn helps to reduce testosterone levels. The fitter you are, the lower your body fat and the better your insulin and glucose control. Less hyperinsulinism means your ovaries are encouraged to produce less testosterone. This can ease your symptoms. Equally important when the symptoms of PCOS result in loss of self-esteem, exercise can help you feel good about yourself and give you a sense of accomplishment. And, once you've made the effort and are feeling the benefits of regular exercise, you are less likely to want to eat unhealthy foods to spoil it.

Exercise has helped me so much. Whether it is yoga, walking, weight-training, running or simply being more active in our daily lives, I think we all need to get more active every day.
Alison, 19

I think I must have tried 1,000 diets – some work for a while and some work well, but as soon as you stop them the weight starts slowly creeping back until it is all back. Even eating like a rabbit (lettuce and sesame seeds) does not cause weight loss. I have come to the conclusion that the only way to really keep it off is by exercising – and unfortunately, with PCOS this often means working harder than anybody else as it takes us three times longer to lose weight.

I find it easier to stay exercising than to diet. And exercising with friends is not only inspiring, it's fun. My advice is to start off really slowly and with something you don't hate – like 10 minutes' cycling on an exercise bike – and build up until you can do an hour. Put on nice music or read a book or watch TV while doing it. Lose a bit of weight first before you start anything more complicated, or else you will either hurt yourself or find you cannot do it and give up. If you are going to the gym, go at off-peak times until you feel more confident – there is nothing more depressing than watching Barbie in a leotard!
Ginney, 36

Recent research continues to confirm that regular, moderate exercise can lower blood-sugar levels and promote insulin efficiency. It also lowers blood pressure and the risk of a heart attack and diabetes. If you have PCOS, exercise may be one of the most effective ways for you to control your symptoms, prevent any need for medication and, of course, lose weight.

Insulin Resistance, Diet and Exercise

If you have PCOS, you have a one-in-three statistical risk of developing insulin resistance – but your real risk increases sharply if you consume a lot of refined carbohydrates and saturated fats, plus insufficient Omega-3 EFAs. But you're not going to wake up one morning to discover that you're suddenly insulin resistant.

Insulin resistance takes years to become severe. If you pay attention to some of the early signs – higher blood pressure and elevated triglyceride and cholesterol levels – when you're in your thirties or forties, you can reverse insulin resistance and stand a good chance of preventing diabetes and coronary heart disease when you're older.

Being overweight increases your risk of developing insulin resistance. But being a thin couch potato is comparable – in terms of your body's metabolic activity – to being fat. Regular exercise, even a daily walk, primes your cells for activity. To get the energy you need for exercise, your body uses insulin to move sugar and fat into cells, where they're burned as fuel. With the increase in insulin activity, sugar levels in the blood decrease. And with less sugar in your blood, your body produces less insulin and becomes more responsive to both sugar and insulin. Insulin sensitivity – the opposite of insulin resistance – goes up, and that's good.

Exercise can help you lose weight because it burns calories. It burns off fat by speeding up your metabolism, and balancing your hormones. And the effects last way beyond your workout. Studies show that fit people burn more calories even while they are resting. It takes more calories to maintain muscle tissue than fat tissue. So the more you exercise, the more your muscles build up and the speedier your metabolism becomes – counteracting the effects of the PCOS weight trap. Don't forget, though, that exercise alone won't do the job. You need to combine exercise with a healthy, balanced diet.

It's Good for You

There's no doubt about it – exercise will do you good if you have PCOS. The American Diabetic Association lists the health benefits of exercise, many of which are particularly relevant for women with PCOS and insulin resistance, including:

❈ You will probably lose weight.
❈ Your blood-sugar levels will be reduced. Exercise lowers your blood-sugar levels by burning it as fuel. Once blood sugar is closer to normal you can be more flexible with your food choices.
❈ Your insulin sensitivity will improve. Regular activity increases a cell's ability to use insulin. With exercise the pancreas does not need to produce as much insulin. Less insulin means less testosterone, which in turn means less acne or hair growth or irregular periods.

❈ Steady exercise for more than 20 minutes allows your muscles to store more glucose (in the form of glucagon), lowering your blood sugar even after you've stopped exercising. Your body will call on these reserves of glucose when your blood-sugar levels become too low.

❈ Other benefits include improved circulation, improved lung function, increased good (HDL) cholesterol, lowered blood pressure, improved sleep, conditioning of the cardiovascular system, increased muscle strength and flexibility, reduced stress and an improved attitude, sense of well-being and quality of life. These will all help to prevent diabetes and heart disease, another reason why exercise really is worth it.

Making exercise a regular part of your life is a great move to make towards a longer, healthier happier life, managing your symptoms and maintaining a healthy body weight. Taking time out of your day for walking, biking or an exercise class could add years – healthy, energetic years – to your future. And you don't have to be stick-thin – even losing a bit of weight or just getting fitter is a good step on the way to better health.

According to Professor Stephen Blair, who studied and produced a report on thousands of Americans at the Cooper Institute in Dallas, being unfit – rather than obesity – is linked with poor health and death. His tests, conducted over several decades, show that physical activity is a more important signpost to health than being overweight. Slim people who are unfit have a death rate double that of those who exercise regularly. Professor Blair hopes this information will encourage everyone to incorporate more activity into their daily lives.

Starting a Fitness Plan

Ideally you should check with your doctor before you begin any exercise routine, especially if you are over 40, have insulin resistance, diabetes, problems related to diabetes (such as eye, kidney or nerve disorders), or high blood pressure.

Once you know it's safe for you to exercise, exercise safely. Listen to your body and use your common sense. Obviously some discomfort and soreness are normal when you are getting fit, but pain isn't normal. Don't overdo it. Set achievable goals for yourself and go at your own pace. Should you feel pain, get short of breath or feel unusually tired, STOP immediately and talk to your doctor.

Be sure to wear loose, comfortable clothing when exercising and make sure your shoes offer you the correct support. Drink plenty of water before, during and after exercise, even if you don't feel thirsty, and have light snacks (fruit, fruit juice, rice crackers) to hand to counteract sudden energy dips.

Make exercise fun. Studies show that exercise drop-outs often punish themselves with exercise routines they don't enjoy. If you know you aren't really going to make use of that expensive exercise equipment, don't buy it. If you hate swimming, don't do it. If the thought of an aerobics class fills you with dread, don't do it. If you find running boring, don't do it. Find an activity you enjoy, so that you can maintain a positive attitude. This can include dancing, horseriding, rambling, etc. – it doesn't have to be a 'traditional' exercise or class.

You might want to ask your partner, a family member or a friend to exercise with you. Again, studies show that when you exercise with other people you are more likely to continue, because you can motivate each other and it is tougher to break the commitment to exercise when you know that others will be working out without you.

Your Routine

Once you've made the decision to start exercising regularly, the next thing you need to know is what exercise goals you should be setting yourself to maximize your chances of weight loss.

A good exercise routine that you can repeat daily, every other day or three times a week, starts with 5 to 10 minutes of gentle warm-up exercises to raise your body temperature and increase your heart rate. This is followed by a period of continuous moderately-paced aerobic conditioning. Aerobic conditioning is essential for heart health and weight control. Aim for 20 to 30 minutes of continuous exercise that works the large muscles of the body and elevates your breathing rate and heart rate. Fast walking is ideal, but you may prefer jogging, swimming or an exercise class.

Walking is particularly good for PCO/S patients because it calms them down. Over the years I have observed that women with PCOS are in high gear most of the time – their minds are constantly racing 90 miles an hour. If I can convince my PCO/S patient to take the time to do it, walking may well be more valuable to her than jogging because the former slows down her mental activity. I think that it is better for this woman to spend an hour walking than 10 minutes running. She needs to give the time to herself – and to recognize that she deserves every minute of it.
Dr Robert Franklin, clinical professor of obstetrics and gynecology at Baylor College of Medicine in Houston, Texas

The key is to give your muscles a good workout and get your heart pumping. As you increase the intensity of your workout, your muscles need more oxygen and your heart beats faster. For optimum weight loss you need to find your 'aerobic training zone'. That means you need to get your heart rate up to 60 to 75 per cent of its maximum capacity (220 minus your age) for around 20 to 45 minutes. If you feel slightly out of breath but not so much that you can't carry on a conversation, you know that you are exercising at the right rate. A cool-down period should follow your aerobic workout.

In addition to this, you need to build in a routine that stretches your muscles and puts your joints through their full range of motion. The best time to stretch is when your muscles are warmed up, after your aerobic workout. Allow about 10 minutes for stretching. Stretching your muscles keeps you flexible. It also lengthens your muscles and strengthens tendons and ligaments. Tai chi and yoga are good ways to improve flexibility and range of motion.

You also need to include some muscle-strengthening activities two or three times a week. Building and maintaining adequate muscle tone will help you burn more calories even when you are not exercising. In addition, good muscle tone will make you look fitter as well as protecting your joints from stress. To strengthen bones and prevent osteoporosis you need to add weight-bearing exercises to your routine.

Walking and bicycling are good weight-bearing exercises, but strength-training is even better. The aim is not to become muscle-bound – you only need to do up to two sets of up 10 repetitions of exercises like press-ups, which work your upper body, and squats, which work your lower body. Fitness clubs offer instruction and weights and weight machines, but if you can't face the gym or it isn't an option you can get the same benefits working out at home with three- to eight-pound dumbbells. An instructional video can also help. To get the most out of weight-training, you need to take the time to know how to perform the exercises with correct technique and form.

Finally, pay attention to your breathing when you exercise. Try to prevent it becoming quick and shallow. In general you should breathe in deeply through your nose and out through your mouth.

You might be reluctant to exercise on a regular basis, but consider this: PCOS puts you at considerable risk of a host of serious health problems, including diabetes, heart disease and obesity – and an exercise programme – even one as simple as walking 15 to 30 minutes a day – could significantly reduce your risk in the coming years. *For women with PCOS, exercise is as important as diet in reducing these risks.*

I never liked exercise. When my doctor suggested a daily exercise programme as part of my treatment for PCOS, I just couldn't see that happening. My husband suggested that I go walking with him. I started slowly. First, short 10-minute walks to the shops and back. Then we extended that to a walk to the shops and the park and back. Then it was a walk to the shops, a walk round the park and back and so on. After a few weeks I was ready to walk even further. In a little over three months I started walking to

work (about a 35-minute walk). Now I walk to work most days and when the weather is beautiful I walk back home again as well at the end of the day. I've lost pounds and feel years younger.
Maddie, 40

Your increased metabolic rate and muscle strength will help you burn calories more efficiently, but there is another reason why exercise is such a great weight loss tool: it can distract you from food and help curb your appetite. Women who exercise regularly find that they don't crave food so often. Apart from taking your mind off food and building self-esteem, regular moderate exercise modifies the activity of the hormones that regulate appetite in a beneficial way, so that you are less likely to get food cravings and/or feel constantly hungry.

WATER RETENTION AND YOUR WEIGHT

Do you feel puffed out and bloated before a period? Do you sometimes feel sluggish and heavy round your ankles, feet and waist? You're not alone. Many women get fluid retention, and it's good to sort out the problem as it can make your weight fluctuate.

Water retention isn't the same as weight gain. When you retain water you do gain weight because your body holds on to water, but in time your body will flush out the water and your weight will stabilize. This isn't always the case with weight gained as fat, which can be permanent unless you make an effort to shift it.

Fluid retention can be a symptom of hormonal imbalance, especially when there is too much oestrogen circulating without the balancing effect of progesterone – often the case for women with PCOS and irregular periods. It can also be the result of excess salt – which causes the body to retain extra fluid to dilute the sodium – and poor vitamin and mineral intake. Many women suffer from PMT fluid retention just before their periods because there is a temporary rise in the body's sodium level.

Food allergies may also be a cause of fluid retention, as the histamine reaction of an allergy causes water to be trapped inside the cells and this can lead to bloating.

Over-the-counter diuretics aren't really a good idea, as they leech valuable nutrients from your body. If you get fluid retention there are a number of steps you can take to help yourself:

Cut down on salt	A decrease in the amount of salt you eat reduces the amount of fluid you gain. Use less in cooking, watch out for hidden salts in your foods and look to other ways of enhancing flavours (see Chapter 2).
Increase your fluid intake	You may try to restrict your fluid intake because you think it will solve the problem of fluid retention. The opposite is true. You need to drink more, not less. Increasing the amount you drink helps your body dilute the salt in your tissues and allows you to excrete more salt and fluid. Aim to drink at least 4 or 5 pints (2 to 3 litres) of water a day. You might find that still water lies in your stomach more easily than sparkling because of the gas in the latter kind.
Reduce your caffeine intake	Caffeine is a diuretic. Fairly soon after drinking it you will find that you need to use the restroom, but it won't ease the bloating because caffeine also hinders the excretion of excess salt and toxins from your body.
Boost your potassium levels	Eating more potassium-rich foods is a good way to bring down your body's sodium level, as the two minerals balance each other out. Reach for those bananas, tomatoes, green leafy vegetables, wholegrains and fresh fruits.

Use grapeseed extract	Studies at the University of Reading have shown the surprising effectiveness of Colladeen, a mix of grapeseed extract, bilberry and cranberry extract, for relief of premenstrual fluid retention.
Take vitamin B_6	When taken as part of a B complex supplement, B_6 is a tried-and-tested remedy for water retention.

You could also try evening primrose oil or a tincture of agnus castus. The aromatherapy oil Roman chamomile, in the bath or a massage, can also help.

WEIGHT-LOSS SUPPLEMENTS

Traditionally, there are three basic approaches to weight loss through nutritional supplements. The first is the use of herbs and nutrients to reduce water retention (see page 199) and speed up metabolism, the second is to use vitamins which have the ability to reduce cholesterol and fat, and the third is the use of natural appetite suppressants.

Below are listed nutritional and herbal supplements that can help you lose weight, but it is important to point out that they can only be effective if you follow a healthy diet according to the guidelines in Chapter 2.

Natural Therapies

Nutritional supplements recommended to aid weight loss include:

Psyllium husks	for fibre, to promote a fuller feeling so you don't eat so much and to clean your colon, which is important for stabilizing weight
Chromium polynicotinate	to reduce sugar cravings
EFAs	for appetite control

Kelp or wheat grass	contain minerals to aid weight loss and calm appetite
Lecithin capsules	help break down fat
Spirulina	a usable protein that can stabilize blood sugar
Vitamin B complex	to combat water retention
Vitamin C	can speed up a slow metabolism
Boron	a US Department of Agriculture study revealed that this trace mineral may speed the burning of calories – raisins and onions are good sources
Amino acids L-ornithine, L-arginine and L-lysine	research has shown that weight loss can be improved with the use of a combination of these, which help release growth hormone when the body is at rest, and builds muscle

Kombucha tea has also shown good results and helps to boost energy.

Also helpful would be a good multivitamin and mineral complex with potassium calcium and zinc, important in the production of energy.

(See Chapter 8 for more information about supplements.)

You should consult a nutritional therapist before taking any of the above supplements. You also need to remember that they won't help you a great deal unless you combine your supplement programme with healthy diet and regular exercise.

Herbal Supplements

Safety first: Before taking any herb or supplement, make sure you consult a doctor or a trained dietician or nutritionist. Certain herbal supplements can be toxic in large doses. For more information see Chapter 8.

Siberian ginseng	helps move fluids and nutrients throughout the body and reduces the stress of adjusting to new eating habits – do not use if you have high blood pressure or heart problems
Aloe vera juice	improves digestion and cleanses the digestive tract
Astralagus	increases energy and improves nutrient absorption – do not use if you have a fever
Fennel	removes mucus and fat from the intestinal tract and is a natural appetite-suppressant
Fenugreek	useful in mobilizing fat within the liver
Hydroxyatriac acid (HCA)	this substance is proving very helpful for weight loss, it can suppress hunger and inhibit the body from turning carbs into fat

Alfalfa, corn silk, dandelion, gravel root, horsetail, hydrangea, hyssop, juniper berries, oat straw, parsley, seawrack, thyme, uva ursi, white ash and yarrow can all be used in tea form for their diuretic properties. If you use these you need to make sure that your diet is packed full of nutrients so you don't get rid of the water-soluble nutrients your body needs to help you lose weight.

Butcher's broom, cardamom, cayenne, cinnamon, garcinia cambogia, ginger, green tea and mustard seed can improve digestion and aid in the metabolism of fat. Do not use cinnamon if you are pregnant.

Bladderwrack, borage seed, hawthorn berry, liquorice root and sarsaparilla stimulate the adrenal glands and improve thyroid function. Use liquorice root only for a maximum of seven days, and do not use it at all if you have high blood pressure.

Guarana and kola nuts are appetite-suppressants. A herbalist can prescribe ephedra, as it suppresses appetite.

Zotrim, which has been launched in the UK by Nature's Remedies, claims to be the first fully herbal weight-management product supported by a full clinical trial, according to a report in the *Journal of Human Nutrition and Dietetics* and *The British Dietetic Association Journal*.[6] A combination of three South American herbs, Zotrim speeds and extends your feeling of fullness and therefore reduces the amount of food you consume. The idea is that this re-educates your stomach to accept less food, which in turn leads to a reduction in overall calories and weight loss.

Another fat-fighting supplement to succeed in trials is conjugated-linoleic acid (CLA). Studies into the effects of CLA on overweight people were carried out at several health centres round the world. According to Dr Michael Pariza, director of the Wisconsin Food Research Institute, the studies were very significant: 'lead[ing] to the idea that CLA can be useful in weight management'.

Acupuncture

Probably the hardest part of dieting to lose weight is overcoming hunger pangs. Acupuncture, properly applied, removes hunger pangs by stimulating the release of the so-called pleasure hormones, endorphins, which are also stimulated by food. Because acupuncture does the work of food in this way, your stomach does not miss it and hunger pangs do not occur. Moreover, specialists in the technique claim that the effects last even after the course of acupuncture is over.

Slimming Drugs

The slimming industry is big business, and if you want to lose weight it can be tempting to try a magic drug or potion. If you have PCOS, however, non-prescription slimming drugs are not a good move. What you need is permanent weight loss; the drawback with slimming drugs is that they don't work in the long term. They either make you lose weight so unnaturally in a few weeks that as soon as you eat normally again it all piles back on again, or they are so far removed from your normal eating habits that you can't stick to them.

Slimming drugs include those based on amphetamines (speed) and thyroxine (animal hormone). These drugs either put you off food or increase your metabolic rate by increasing your heart rate. If you have PCOS, these drugs should be avoided completely. They will make your body behave in a strange way and make your symptoms even worse. All slimming drugs have adverse side-effects that are potentially harmful to your health.

Prescribable slimming drugs, like Xenical (orlistat) and Sibutramine (reductil) can be a helpful option but only as part of a healthy diet and lifestyle. The priority for women with PCOS is to establish long-term healthy eating patterns that are practical and sustainable for the rest of their lives. Sally Wharmby and Claire Mellors, Senior Dietitians, Queens Medical Centre, Nottingham

Having said this, if your doctor feels that your weight carries with it a serious threat to your health unless you take a short-term dieting drug, then it can be a useful step on the way to changing your diet and lifestyle – as long as you don't rely on it for long-term health but see it instead as very much a short-term solution.

Reductil

The drug Reductil has been described as a revolutionary step in the fight against excess weight gain. The National Institute of Clinical Excellence has recommended that the drug should be available on the NHS in the UK. The drug works by 'tricking' your brain into making you feel full. Unlike existing drugs for obesity such as Xenical (which prevents fat from being absorbed by the body), Reductil has not been found to have significant side-effects. Over three million people around the world have taken Reductil, also called Sibutramine. A recent study suggested that patients lost an average of 20 lb over six months.

Medication can improve the chances of success when dieting. But it is important to point out that any supplement or drug is most effective for weight loss only when combined with a healthy diet (see Chapter 2) and an exercise plan (see Chapter 7).

GETTING MOTIVATED

One of the biggest problems in losing weight is motivation. It's all very well saying it should be done for the good of your health and to keep your symptoms at bay, but is this enough?

Everybody knows that slimming means more exercise and a healthy diet, but 95 per cent of people (according to a Psychology Today survey) still fail to achieve permanent weight loss by traditional methods because they can't maintain their motivation.
Fitness trainer Pete Cohen, who runs nationwide weight-loss workshops and courses (Lighten Up) in the UK

I'm great at starting diets, but not so good at sticking at them. If I don't see results right in the first week or two I get demotivated and give up, but if I do see results quickly, say I lose weight and I get a regular period, I'm so delighted that I forget all about the diet and the weight piles back on.
Denise, 39

I guess I just get bored with thinking about what I should eat all the time and how it will affect my symptoms. At the start of every month I promise myself that this time I'm going to last the course, but life gets in the way and I never do. Even if I have seen results and I've lost weight, all my efforts just seem to dwindle to nothing.
Sinead, 33

You may want to lose weight, but do you want it enough to make it happen? You may fear making changes that may overwhelm you. We all have an instinct to avoid pain and seek pleasure. Your current lifestyle may not be that healthy, but at least it is familiar. PCOS isn't life-threatening in the short term, and for most of us the present has to get really uncomfortable for us to be jolted into change, so if you are reading this book and still can't get motivated, is there anything that can help?

Write It Down

Keeping a food diary works well because it focuses you. It makes what you are doing real and makes you really think about whether your diet is helping your symptoms or just making them worse. A food diary also reminds you of your goal and gives you a feeling of control.
Holly, 40

Start today by writing down everything you eat and drink. You might also want to note down how much time you spend exercising. Don't make any changes in the first week, just start becoming aware of your eating and exercise routines. At the end of the week, review your diary and see where positive changes can be made for the weeks ahead.

Control is one way a diary can help, but writing things down is also about awareness and encouraging you to notice what you are doing. You can't change habits you are not aware of.

In addition to keeping a food diary, you might want to consider drawing up a contract with yourself to change. In it you could agree that from this moment on you will make the changes to your eating and exercise routines that can help make you slimmer, fitter and healthier. A contract with yourself may sound odd, but studies show that writing down your goals and aspirations makes them more real and helps you stay focused on achieving them.

Identify Triggers

Are there certain kinds of foods you can't live without? Are there certain places, like bars or parties, or certain emotions, like fear and sadness, which make you want to overeat? The important thing is to become aware of these triggers. Once you become more aware of them, you can start to deal with them.

If you get the urge to eat, try to ride it out. Food cravings peak and subside like waves. When you get the urge to eat, tell yourself you can satisfy that urge to eat if you want. Then wait a few minutes. This ensures that your eating is conscious, not compulsive. Most cravings last only a few minutes. Try doing something to distract yourself. Also remember that food addiction is the same as any other addiction: one bite will never be enough. If you ultimately decide you really do want the food, then decide how much is reasonable and enjoy it. Chew it slowly and savour the taste.

Find out what causes your cravings. If you get a strong urge to snack while watching TV, try reading a book, drinking a glass of water or doing something else while you watch (riding on an exercise bike, doing some needlework, etc.) instead. If your cravings are triggered by being in the kitchen, go for a walk or do some gardening. If you are out shopping, try to avoid cafes and restaurants.

Join a Support Group

You may be the kind of woman who enjoys setting goals and achieving them by yourself, but even so, a slimming or PCOS support group can be helpful. Make sure, though, that if you join a weight-loss group your leader or individual dieting coach has an understanding of PCOS and the added complications and frustrations it can bring. PCOS support groups can offer you contacts, friends or advice.

You may prefer to get the support you need from partners, friends and family who know about your condition. But if being weighed in front of others at a weight-loss group, talking to friends and family, or contacting others via support groups doesn't appeal, weight-loss coaching services which encourage people to lose weight over the phone might interest you. The anonymous arena of a telephone conference call can encourage you to share your experiences openly. You will be encouraged, supported and coached to help you stick to basic, healthy weight-loss principles and achieve steady, sustainable weight loss. The aim is to help you think like a naturally slim person so you will never have to diet again.

(For more information about support groups and diet coaching on the phone, see Chapter 12.)

THE ROAD TO SUCCESS

Knowing that you need to lose weight or wishing that you could lose weight isn't the same as making the decision to lose weight. Motivational techniques such as visualization help you get in touch with what you really want, and remind you that nothing in life worth having comes easy. Such techniques can bring focus and commitment to your weight-loss plan.

Of utmost importance to women with PCOS is the realization that you need to follow a diet and exercise programme you can live with for the rest of your life. We've seen that fasting and fad diets are not the answer. It sounds harsh, but once you see that there is no quick fix you can start to change your whole body image, partly through a healthy diet and regular exercise programme and medication if needed, but mainly through understanding. You need to understand that excess weight will affect your hormones and make your PCOS symptoms worse.

Losing weight won't be easy, but you mustn't use PCOS as an excuse to give up. There will be times when you feel that you are failing and want to give up:

I've lost count of the number of times I've tried to lose weight. I always end up overindulging, my symptoms get worse and I feel like I have let myself down.
Clare, 31

It's important that you expect setbacks. Make weight loss your goal, if you have weight to lose, but don't give up or punish yourself if you overindulge on the odd occasion. People who try but fail are twice as likely to succeed next time. A lot depends on your attitude. Thinking in terms of failure won't help you. Turn your thinking around. There is no such thing as failure – only setbacks on the road to success.

If you have tried everything and you still can't lose weight, the information in Chapter 11 may help. Losing weight is often complicated, tied in as it often can be with guilt, comfort relationships with food, lack of self-esteem, the hectic pace of life, low moods and exasperation with PCOS symptoms. In Chapter 11 we'll explore how food, eating patterns and weight-management are so often linked to emotions, and how you can move towards healthier attitudes to food.

THE PILL AND YOUR WEIGHT

If you are taking the oral contraceptive pill to manage your symptoms and/or because it is your choice of contraception, you may be wondering if that is making it harder for you to lose weight.

Although many doctors don't think the Pill is to blame, many women who start taking it do say they notice weight gain and feelings of bloatedness when they are taking this form of medication, and the British Medical Association's *Official Guide to Medicines and Drugs* does list weight gain as a possible side-effect. We've also seen that the Pill can make women insulin resistant. The BMA guide says, 'Oestrogens may also trigger the onset of diabetes mellitus in susceptible people, or aggravate blood-sugar control in diabetic women.'[7] Whether it is excess weight that causes insulin resistance or the increased insulin resistance that causes weight gain is not clear. The fact is both can occur, and both are associated with a worsening of PCOS symptoms.

There are health risks associated with being on the Pill and being overweight. Synthetic oestrogens in the Pill can increase the drive towards insulin resistance, a precursor state to diabetes. There is also the much publicized risk of blood clots, as well as high blood pressure and perhaps breast cancer. Listed alongside smoking as one of the factors which increases all these risks is being overweight. So for women with PCOS who have weight problems, being on the Pill could be taking a dangerous risk with your health if you are not following a healthy-eating, no-smoking, healthy-living plan and regularly communicating with your healthcare professional.

Should I Take the Pill?

The Pill is a good form of contraception, but if you are taking the Pill as your preferred choice of contraception you should be aware of the risks if you have PCOS. If you are taking the Pill as a treatment for irregular periods, you might think about making diet and lifestyle changes before resorting to the Pill. And however much the symptoms of PCOS improve when you are on the Pill, don't forget that the Pill only masks the symptoms of PCOS, it doesn't cure them. It can only ever be a temporary solution for PCOS. The permanent solution is to make healthy diet and lifestyle changes, with or without medication – and, of course, to lose weight if you have weight to lose.

If, however, you are aware of the risks and want to stay on the Pill for the time being you need to know which brands may affect PCOS and your weight the most.

Which Brand Is Right for Me?

Oral contraceptives come in two basic types – oestrogen-containing combined and phased oral contraceptives, and progesterone-only contraceptives.

The combined oral contraceptive pill is the most widely prescribed because it is the most reliable. There are many different products available. They are divided into three groups according to their oestrogen content (please note: UK brand names may differ from those used in the US):

1 Low-oestrogen brands such as Mercilon, Minulet, Ovran, Femodene, Loestrin and Ovranette
2 Medium-dose brands such as Brevinor, Cilest, Norimin and Ovysmen
3 High-dose brands such as Norinyl-1, Ortho Novin 1/50 and Ovran

The newest form of contraception is a pack of pills divided into two or three groups or phases. Each phase contains a different proportion of oestrogen and progesterone. The aim is to provide a hormonal balance that closely resembles the fluctuations of a normal menstrual cycle. UK brand names include BiNovum, Logynon, Synphase, Triadene, TriMinulet, TriNordial and TriNovum.

Progesterone-only pills are slightly less reliable and must be taken at exactly the same time each day to have effect. UK brand names include Femulen, Micronor, Micoval, Neogest, Norgeston and Noriday.

You might think that progesterone-only pills may be the best form of oral contraceptive for women with PCOS, as they lack the oestrogen-related side-effects and risks and the drive towards insulin resistance. Yet some women find that progesterone-only pills or pills with low doses of oestrogen don't properly suppress PCOS symptoms, and even seem to make symptoms worse. One study at the University of Southern California Medical School found that the contraceptives identified as producing the greatest risk of diabetes, which women who have PCOS already have a risk of developing, were progestin-only pills (progestin is a synthetic form or progesterone), along with oestrogen-progestin combinations containing the strongest progestins.[8] However, a study from Harvard Medical School placed the blame for this increased risk not on the Pill but on excess weight. Of the contraceptives studied, the combination pill containing norethindrome appeared to be the safest and did not increase the risk of diabetes.

In terms of the androgenic effects of progesterone in oral contraceptives, certain brands are likely to make symptoms of PCOS worse, according to Dr Helen Mason, senior Lecturer in Reproductive Endocrinology at St George's Hospital Medical School, London:

Norethisterone is the most androgenic, [found] in Brevinor, Loestrin, Trinovum and should be avoided. The next most androgenic is levonorgestrel, [found] in Logynon, Microgynon, Ovran, and then Desogestrel, [found] in Marvelon. It seems that cyproterene acetate [found] in Dianette is the least [androgenic], and as a result it is commonly prescribed for hirsutism. If you have PCOS and suffer from acne or hirsutism, Dianette is probably your best choice.

Cilest is another brand to try if body hair increases. If you are prone to acne, you need to go for contraceptive pills with the new progesterones which are less active on skin receptors. Minulet, Femodene, Ovysmen or Brevinor have a lower progesterone effect and are less likely to cause acne. Dr Adam Balen, Consultant Obstetrician and Gynaecologist and Specialist in Reproductive Medicine and Surgery at Leeds General Infirmary, UK, is currently researching a new pill, which he believes may take over from Dianette as the preferred choice of oral contraceptive for women with PCOS symptoms such as acne. 'The pill is called Yasmin – to be released in the UK in April 2002 and we are researching to see if it is better.'

Your Individual Needs

Weight gain tends to be most common in higher-dose pills, which are starting to become a thing of the past. Switching to lower doses may help, but even low-dose oestrogen pills can cause water retention, and progesterone can still increase appetite. If you are concerned about weight gain, pills containing the most modern progesterones (such as Femodene) reduce the risk of weight gain – but you need to check with your doctor that this is the right pill for you and your symptoms.

Don't forget that weight gain may not be related to the Pill at all. You may simply be eating more. Many women feel that now they are on the Pill they are bound to put on weight, and then let themselves go a bit and eat more than usual. It's tempting to blame the Pill for weight gain, but if you are on a low-dose pill there is no reason why, with careful attention to your diet and regular exercise, you shouldn't be able to manage your weight.

Experiences with oral contraceptives can vary from woman to woman:

I'm taking a combined pill at the moment. I used to take the progesterone-only one for about five years, but it isn't strong enough for me now. I seemed to be bleeding all the time. I switched about a year ago and have stopped growing hair where I don't want it and my cycles are regular. Fingers crossed this pill is controlling my symptoms well.
Chloe, 23

I took the new phased pills for a year but then I put on a lot of weight and my symptoms got worse. My doctor switched me back to a combined pill and I lost a bit of weight but my periods got too heavy and I became anaemic. I've since switched to two different types of pill and neither has really helped.
Kim, 30

How Long Should I Stay on the Pill?

It's impossible to say how long you should stay on the Pill, as each woman is different. You need to discuss this carefully with your doctor. Some women with PCOS feel fine on the Pill, but others experience unpleasant side-effects. Some women gain weight, others don't. There is no uniform recommendation for the right medication to manage your symptoms.

The best advice is to proceed with caution if you are on an oral contraceptive, and to monitor things carefully. Keep a written record and make sure your doctor monitors you closely, too. If you think the Pill is making you feel worse, tell your doctor right away. If you have taken a pill for several months and think you are reacting poorly to it, ask to switch to another type. You may also find that after taking one brand of pill for several years your symptoms seem to be returning, perhaps as a result of increased insulin resistance. If you think the Pill is triggering weight gain, ask your doctor for advice.

Essential Nutrients When You Are on the Pill

According to a 1984 study in the *Journal of Reproductive Medicine*, 'Women who take OCs [oral contraceptives] and have adequate diets need little or no supplemental vitamins'[9] – but this is assuming that everyone eats a highly nutritious and balanced diet. Nor does it take into account the increased nutritional needs of women with PCOS. The Pill can leech valuable supplements and nutrients, as well as alter your vitamin and mineral levels.[10] Studies suggest that the Pill lowers levels of vitamin B_1, B_2 and B_6 in the blood. Folic acid, vitamin B_{12}, vitamin C and vitamin E are also affected by the Pill. Levels of vitamin A and iron increase slightly, as do levels of copper – which isn't necessarily a good thing as high copper levels can increase the risk of high blood pressure. Zinc is perhaps the most important mineral that can be affected by the Pill. The Pill is known to change a woman's capacity to absorb zinc. You need sufficient levels of zinc to maintain a healthy reproductive system and hormonal balance.

If you are on the Pill, on top of your basic healthy diet it is wise to supplement extra vitamin B complex to help your liver break down synthetic hormones effectively. You might also consider taking a zinc mineral supplement.

We also know that the Pill can kill friendly bacteria in your gut, which can cause digestive problems such as IBS. Live yogurt, which contains natural probiotics, should be on your daily menu to replenish the bacterial balance. If you are dairy intolerant you can buy fruit-based drinks with live bacterial cultures from healthfood stores.

The Pill can also lower levels of good cholesterol and increase levels of bad cholesterol, so you need to ensure that you eat foods that promote good cholesterol – something which will also help to reduce your risk of heart disease.

A to Z of Useful Supplements and How to Use Them

A healthy diet is always the basis of good health, but because so many factors are involved in PCOS, taking supplements may be extremely beneficial.

While you are working on your diet, supplements and herbs can be extremely useful for correcting PCOS. If you have been using the Pill to regulate your periods, you may have an even greater imbalance between a number of key nutrients. Correcting this imbalance will go a long way towards treating the root cause of the problem. Making changes and adding supplements to your diet will help to control blood sugar, while herbs go one step further, targeting any problems involving hormone balance. Herbs can also be very beneficial in encouraging the functions of the liver in order to make sure that it is metabolizing the hormones efficiently and then eliminating them.
Dr Marilyn Glenville, nutritionist and natural fertility specialist

Eating healthily and gently detoxing your diet are the priority if you have PCOS. Supplements should be seen as a way for you to support these positive changes. A nutritionist would typically recommend a good multivitamin and mineral, along with an antioxidant complex and essential fatty acid supplement for women with PCOS. After that, the herbs and supplements we recommend depend very much on a woman's individual symptoms. If she wants to fall pregnant, if she wants to lose weight, if she wants to see an improvement in her acne, and so on.
Dr Adam Carey, nutritionist

The term 'supplement' covers a broad range of vitamins, minerals and plant extracts which should be taken to complement – not replace – a healthy, balanced diet. The most popular supplement is the multivitamin/mineral, which most nutritionists regard as a good insurance policy and which can be taken long term.

If you have PCOS you can't afford to be deficient in any of the essential nutrients, so on top of your healthy diet you should consider taking a multivitamin and mineral supplement containing vitamins A, D, E, C, B_1, B_2, B_3, B_5, B_6, B_{12}, folic acid, calcium, magnesium, iron, zinc, chromium, selenium and manganese. You cannot fit all the above vitamins and minerals into one tablet, so a qualified nutritionist will probably recommend two or more tablets a day to meet your requirements. The bulkiest nutrients are vitamin C, calcium and magnesium which are often inadequately supplied in a multivitamin and mineral and may need to be taken separately.

Any herbs you may take in addition to your multivitamin and mineral should match your unique symptoms and needs.

Remember that *supplements are not a substitute for eating a healthy diet.*

It is best to take most of your supplements as early in the day as possible. You need to take your supplements regularly to see and feel improvements. Ideally you should have a nutritional therapist or herbalist make up a prescription for you.

BE CAUTIOUS

Including the right supplements and herbs in your diet may help your body adapt by restoring and maintaining hormonal imbalance and improving your symptoms. Many supplements designed to support female health are likely to be safe and beneficial. However, large amounts of any herb or dietary supplement should be taken only under the guidance of a doctor or a qualified nutritional consultant or herbalist.

If you are on any kind of medication, have high blood pressure, diabetes or insulin resistance, again you should take herbs and supplements only under professional guidance. If you are pregnant, it is crucial that you seek the advice of your doctor or a trained professional. Many of the supplements listed in this chapter are contraindicated when pregnant. (For useful general guidelines on contraindications with prescription medications, contact the NutriCentre – their website address is www.nutricentre.com.)

The herbs and supplements listed below are those which have been used with varying degrees of success by some women with PCOS. If you do decide to take herbs in addition to your multivitamin and mineral, it is important that you check with your doctor or a qualified expert that they are safe for you to take. There is generally no danger of using herbs alongside nutrient supplements such as vitamins and minerals. But before you start self-medicating, get the all-clear from a professional first.

The aim of the nutritional guidelines outlined in this book is to ensure that you make safe and sensible changes in your diet which will improve your symptoms and well-being. They are not intended to replace the individually-tailored advice of a qualified doctor, nutritionist or herbalist.

Read the Label

Not all supplements are true to their labels, so it is not always best to buy the cheapest. Reputable companies, however, should give you a list of all the ingredients on the label. For most supplements the ingredients have to be listed in order of weight, with the ingredient present in the highest quality heading the list. This can be confusing as often the chemical name of the nutrient is used instead of the common vitamin name. This can be a bit confusing; here are some of the alternative names for nutrients:

A	retinol or beta carotene
B_1	thiamine
B_2	riboflavin

B_3	niacin
B_5	pantothenic acid
B_6	pyridoxine
B_{12}	cyanocobalamine
C	ascorbic acid
D	ergocalciferol, cholecalciferol
E	d (1) alpha tocopherol
Folic acid	folate

When you know which nutrient is which, look for the amount provided by each daily dose. Some supplements state this in terms of two tablets daily. The amount supplied will be given in milligrams (mg) or micrograms (mcg or /μg). Most countries are now switching to /μg as the symbol of micrograms, which are a thousandth of a milligram.

As for minerals, what you want to know is the amount of the actual mineral, *not* the amount of the mineral compound it is added to. Most reputable companies make this easy for you by stating something like 'zinc amino acid chelate (providing 5 mg of zinc) 50 mg' – which means you are getting 5 mg of actual zinc.

Supplements can also contain other ingredients necessary to make them stick together to form a tablet. Fillers, lubricants and coatings are added. Unfortunately many tablets also have artificial colouring and flavouring added, too. Examples of fillers and binders which are perfectly acceptable include: dicalcium phosphate, cellulose, gum arabic, silica, zein, Brazil wax, alginic acid, sodium alginate, calcium or magnesium sterate.

Some fillers and binders, such as sterate, are made from animal fat, so if you are a vegetarian or vegan you may have to check for products that state, 'suitable for vegetarians or vegans' on the labels.

Many of the better supplements will also declare that they are free from sugar and gluten. If you are allergic to milk or yeast, check that the tablet is free from lactose and yeast. B vitamins can be derived from yeast, so be careful. If in doubt contact the company and ask for an independent list of the ingredients. Good manufacturers will be happy to supply this.

You really are better off paying a little more for quality supplements from reputable companies which emphasize quality control and which, if asked, can supply you with independent analyses of their products. It's better to have half a quality tablet than the full dose of a mediocre one.

Herbal treatments work for me, but what works for me may not work for you. You need to figure out what they actually can do for you before taking a whole bunch of herbs. How much of what herb you need will vary greatly from one woman with PCOS to another. Not everyone has the same symptoms to be treated, either, so I would suggest that you base any treatment you approach on either tests done by your doc (good starting point) or connect, like I did, with a herbalist or naturopathic physician. Also, herbs take a lot more time to affect the body compared to drugs, so you must be prepared to wait several months to see results, depending upon your condition.

Having said that, both vitex and saw palmetto would probably be a good place to start. (Also watching the kind of carbohydrates you eat can truly help regulate symptoms.) Progesterone is probably still a good idea, but, if you can, try to make sure you choose a brand which doesn't give you unpleasant side-effects like depression, heavy periods and headaches (in my experience).
Grace, 40

A TO Z OF HERBS AND SUPPLEMENTS FOR WOMEN WITH PCOS

Agnus Castus (Chasteberry)

helps with

- ❀ acne
- ❀ breast tenderness
- ❀ infertility
- ❀ irregular or absent periods
- ❀ hormone imbalance

❋ mood swings
❋ PMS symptoms
❋ water retention

This is a popular herb which grows in Mediterranean countries and central Asia. It normalizes the function of the pituitary gland, which controls and balances your hormones by stimulating the release of luteinizing hormone (LH) so that progesterone levels are increased in relation to oestrogen.

The herb has been used for centuries by women who don't produce enough oestrogen in the second half of their cycle. In one study, 48 women diagnosed with infertility took agnus castus for three months.[1] Seven became pregnant and 25 of them regained normal progesterone levels.

Agnus castus is also thought to help acne, fluid retention and other symptoms of PMS. The most-quoted studies were conducted in Germany and involved more than 1,500 women participants. Physicians and patients both reported 90 per cent relief from PMS symptoms after taking agnus castus for one month.[2]

Agnus castus is an adaptogen, which means that whether you suffer from a low level of one hormone or an excess of another you can take agnus castus and achieve normal levels. Side-effects include minor gastrointestinal upset and a mild rash with itching.

Available from health food stores, herbalists and nutritional therapists, agnus castus is usually marketed under the name Vitex. It comes in several forms and should be taken over a period of several months to determine efficacy.

If you have a hormonal imbalance or your cycles are irregular then it might be worth taking the herb agnus castus over a few months as it is a good balancing herb. Buy an organic tincture of agnus castus and take 1 teaspoon three times a day for three or four months.
Dr Marilyn Glenville

Caution
Before taking this herb, check with your doctor that it is safe to do so. If depression is one of your PMS symptoms, you should probably avoid agnus castus. Some research suggests that PMS with depression may be caused by excess progesterone, and agnus castus is thought to raise progesterone levels. Those with high levels of luteinizing hormone should probably avoid this herb as well. Pregnant women are not advised to use this herb.

Aloe Vera

helps with

- ❋ acne
- ❋ diabetes
- ❋ digestive disorders
- ❋ dry skin
- ❋ insulin resistance
- ❋ obesity

This plant is known for its healing effect and is used in many cosmetic and hair products. There are over 200 different types of aloe grown in dry regions around the world.

Aloe vera is commonly known as a skin healer, moisturizer and softener. Taken internally, 98–99 per cent pure aloe vera is known to aid in the healing of stomach disorders and colon problems. Regular use will keep the colon clean and stools normal.

In a study at the Mahidol Medical University and Hospital, Bangkok, 49 diabetes sufferers were given 1 tablespoon of aloe vera juice twice daily. Blood-sugar levels normalized after two weeks.[3]

Caution
Allergy, though rare, can occur. Before using, apply a small amount behind the ear or on the underarm. If stinging or a rash develops, do not use.

Alpha-lipoic Acid

helps with

- ❄ diabetes
- ❄ insulin resistance
- ❄ obesity

A number of micronutrients help insulin efficiently move glucose into the body's cells. If you think of your body's cells as engines, refined carbohydrates provide plenty of high-grade fuel. But you also need spark plugs to ignite the fuel. One of the most promising of these biological spark plugs is alpha-lipoic acid.

A natural constituent of the body's cells, alpha-lipoic plays a fundamental role in converting glucose to energy. Researchers have found it can lower and stabilize glucose levels and, in Germany, alpha-lipoic acid is sold as a drug for the treatment of diabetic polyneuropathy, a type of severe nerve pain. Stephan Jacob MD of the University of Tübingen, Germany, studied 74 diabetes patients given at least 600 mg of alpha-lipoic acid supplements daily. The alpha-lipoic acid stimulated insulin activity, which safely lowered and stabilized glucose levels. It also made the patients more insulin sensitive and increased their glucose tolerance – both positive changes.

As antioxidants go, alpha-lipoic acid is also extremely important, according to researchers at the University of California. In 1988 they discovered that it was one of the most potent and versatile antioxidants (see below). It also helps recycle vitamin E and other antioxidants such as vitamin C and CoQ10.

If your diet is high in antioxidants or you take an antioxidant complex, supplementation with alpha-lipoic acid probably isn't necessary unless advised by a doctor.

Antioxidant Complex

helps with

- ❋ acne
- ❋ diabetes
- ❋ infertility (especially zinc, selenium)
- ❋ insulin resistance
- ❋ irregular or absent periods (especially zinc, selenium)

Certain vitamins and minerals are known as antioxidants. They are important for skin health and for reducing the risk of diabetes and cancer in all women with PCOS. More research is needed as to whether antioxidants can prevent diabetes, but scientists do agree that these essential nutrients, so abundant in fruits and vegetables, promote good health in countless ways, and may be particularly important for women with PCOS who are insulin resistant[4] and at risk of developing diabetes.[5]

Antioxidants inhibit the harmful chemical process known as oxidation by neutralizing free radicals. Free radicals are the unstable, highly reactive and potentially harmful molecules formed in the body by exposure to sunlight, cigarette smoke and environmental pollutants. Without intervention, free radicals wreak damage at a cellular level and this accelerates the ageing process (which shows up on your skin in the form of wrinkles) and compromises the immune system. In addition to diabetes, conditions as varied as cancer, joint disease, asthma, senility and poor vision have all been linked to free radical damage.

Other antioxidants include alpha-lipoic acid, the vitamin-like substance co-enzyme Q10, and various other enzymes and flavonoids. If you exercise a lot, and are exposed to a lot of stress and chemical pollutants, it might be wise to add an antioxidant complex to your supplement programme. This should contain reasonable amounts of the following antioxidants: vitamins A, C, E, beta carotene, zinc, selenium, iron, copper, manganese and the amino acids glutathione and cysteine, plus phytonutrient antioxidants such as bilberry extract, pycnogenol or grapeseed extract.

If you are eating a healthy diet and taking a multivitamin and mineral supplement you may not need to take additional antioxidants unless advised by a doctor or nutritional therapist. Antioxidants are abundant in fruits, vegetables and sprouted grains, so make sure you include plenty of these foods in your diet.

Astralagus

helps with

- ❈ fainting and/or dizziness
- ❈ fatigue
- ❈ obesity

Astralagus is a tonic herb, frequently used in Traditional Chinese Medicine, which aids adrenal function and boosts your immunity and general health. It is thought to increase energy and improve nutrient absorption. It also has a metabolism-increasing effect. Take up to three 400 mg capsules daily.

Caution
Astralagus should not be taken when you have a fever.

Bitter Melon

helps with

- ❈ diabetes
- ❈ insulin resistance

Also known as *Momordica charentia*, this herb has been traditionally used by Ayurvedic healers to treat Type II diabetes. Numerous studies show that it can normalize elevated blood levels. Indian researchers claim that it may boost the production of insulin, the key hormone in the breakdown of sugar. Bitter melon also holds great promise as a cancer treatment. Fresh bitter melon is available and it is also sold in extracts and capsules. Women with PCOS and insulin resistance or diabetes should take as directed by an Ayurvedic practitioner.

Black Cohosh

helps with

- ❋ breast tenderness
- ❋ depression
- ❋ hot flushes/flashes
- ❋ menstrual cramps
- ❋ irregular or absent periods
- ❋ irritability

The roots and herbs of the forest plant black cohosh provide a phytoestrogen and a biologically active ingredient that dilates blood vessels. The phytoestrogen can relieve many symptoms associated with PMS and the menopause. Also known as black snakeroot, it is thought to lower blood pressure and cholesterol levels and improve thyroid function.

In the journal *Whole Foods*, Dr Judy Christianson stated that in a recent double-blind study, Remifemin (popular brand name for black cohosh in the US) was more effective than Premarin in dealing with menopausal symptoms such as anxiety, depression and vaginal dryness. No studies have been conducted on women with PCOS, but as the herb has a balancing effect on the hormonal system it is often prescribed by medical herbalists for women with PCOS who have irregular cycles and PMS symptoms.

Caution
This herb promotes menstruation and should be avoided during pregnancy. It has other potential side-effects, and should only be used under the supervision of an educated practitioner.

Blue Cohosh

helps with

- ✳ anxiety
- ✳ irregular or absent periods
- ✳ irritability
- ✳ mental fogginess

This herb is thought to be a uterine tonic, suggesting it can increase the muscle tone of a weak uterus. It should be used under the supervision of a professional, and not be used at all in the first two trimesters of pregnancy.

Brewer's Yeast

helps with

- ✳ fainting and/or dizziness
- ✳ fatigue
- ✳ food cravings
- ✳ insulin resistance
- ✳ mental fogginess
- ✳ nervousness

Brewer's yeast is grown on hops, a bitter herb that is also used as an ingredient in beer. It is rich in basic nutrients, especially B vitamins, as well as essential fatty acids, iron, vitamin A, C and E and the minerals chromium, selenium, manganese, copper, iron and zinc – all crucial nutrients for women with PCOS.

The yeast may be consumed in juice or water and is a good energy-booster between meals.

Caution
Do not take brewer's yeast if you get or have thrush (*Candida albicans*).

Burdock

helps with

✿ acne
✿ excess hair

Burdock increases circulation to the skin, which helps detoxify skin tissues and improves nutrition to skin cells. It is also a time-honoured blood- and liver-cleanser and assists in the removal of toxins through the kidneys, ultimately aiding in the balancing of the high levels of testosterone associated with acne and excess hair. Take 1 capsule or 30 drops of tincture with each meal for up to two months.

Vitamin B Complex

helps with

✿ acne (B_6)
✿ adrenal health (B_5)
✿ anxiety (B_1)
✿ depression (B_1, B_6)
✿ diabetes (B_1, B_3, B_6)
✿ excess hair
✿ fainting and/or dizziness
✿ fatigue (B_3, B_5)
✿ food cravings
✿ hair loss
✿ hormonal imbalance (B_6)
✿ infertility (B_6)
✿ insulin resistance (B_1, B_3, B_6)
✿ irregular or absent periods (B_6, B_{12})
✿ irritability
✿ lack of energy (B_3)
✿ liver health
✿ mental fogginess

❈ mood swings (B$_6$)
❈ obesity
❈ poor memory (B$_1$)
❈ skin and hair problems (biotin)
❈ sleep problems/insomnia
❈ water retention (B$_6$)

'The B vitamins are very important in helping to correct the symptoms of PCOS,' says Dr Marilyn Glenville, who treats women with PCOS at her London and Tunbridge Wells Clinics.

B vitamins are essential for healthy liver function and proper digestion and absorption. If you have PCOS it is important that your liver is functioning well. The liver is the body's waste-disposal system not only for toxins and waste products but also for hormones. If your liver isn't functioning well, you may get an accumulation of old hormones left over from each menstrual cycle. The liver deactivates the old hormones and renders them harmless. B vitamins help your body carry out this process.

Research has also shown that giving women vitamin B$_6$ increases their fertility. In one study, 12 out of 14 women who had been trying to conceive for seven years conceived after taking vitamin B$_6$ daily for six months.[6]

Since several of the B vitamins figure strongly in blood-sugar control and energy production, if you want to take extra B vitamins it is advisable to take a supplement of vitamin B-complex rather than separate supplements of each B vitamin. Stress, poor diet, over-exercising, smoking, caffeine, alcohol, exposure to environmental toxins, and in some cases the Pill, can all deplete the body of essential B vitamins. Supplement with one 50 mg vitamin B Complex capsule daily.

Chromium

helps with

- ❀ acne
- ❀ diabetes
- ❀ food cravings
- ❀ insulin resistance
- ❀ mood swings
- ❀ obesity

Chromium is an essential mineral which helps lower glucose levels. Many women with PCOS don't consume enough chromium in their diet and this leaves them depleted. In this depleted state their insulin may not be able to exert its usual effect, making them vulnerable to insulin resistance and diabetes. Several well-documented studies have shown that supplementing with chromium may improve blood-sugar control in insulin-resistant individuals.[7]

Rich food sources of chromium include brewer's yeast (see page 227), wholemeal bread, rye bread, chilli, oysters, chicken, cornmeal, bananas, carrots, oranges, green beans, cabbage, mushrooms and strawberries. Egg yolks, pork and liver also contain this mineral, but you wouldn't want to include these in your diet on a regular basis since excess amounts would raise your cholesterol. Taking chromium supplements in the short term while making dietary changes may also be useful.

In addition to its role in regulating blood sugar, chromium can help you maintain healthy levels of HDL (the good cholesterol). Chromium is also the most widely researched mineral used in the treatment of the overweight. One study shows that people who took chromium picolinate over a 10-week period lost an average of 1.9 kg while those on a placebo lost only 0.2 kg.[8]

Studies are under way to determine which type of chromium supplement is best for women with PCOS. The organic, chelated forms – such as chromium picolinate (chromium bonded to the amino acid picolinate) and chromium polynicotinate (chromium bonded to niacin) are better absorbed than standard chromium supplements. Most people who supplement with chromium take 50 to 200 mcg a day. Up to 1,000 mcg is considered safe.

Cinnamon

helps with

❄ insulin resistance
❄ obesity

A herb widely used in cookery, cinnamon is a warming digestive and circulatory stimulant. It is also thought to make fat cells more responsive to insulin, helping them to metabolize glucose.

The US Department of Agriculture Nutritional Research Center has reported that cinnamon, cloves, turmeric (see page 255) and bay leaves help stimulate insulin activity. Of these, cinnamon was found to be the most potent. Only a little cinnamon, such as a small amount sprinkled on toast, can do the trick. A dash of cinnamon or half a teaspoon with every meal on any number of appropriate dishes may help keep blood-sugar levels in check.

Caution
Do not use large amounts during pregnancy.

CLA

helps with

❄ diabetes
❄ overweight

CLA (Conjugated Linoleic Acid) is a weight-loss supplement which may help women with PCOS if they have weight to lose. It contains the right kind of fat which can help your body regulate fat and metabolize protein. Numerous studies have shown that CLA can offer many health benefits, and in particular can reduce the amount of body fat while increasing muscle.

It is very difficult to get enough CLA from the food you eat. This is because many of us avoid foods that are rich in CLA, such as red meat, lamb and dairy produce, because they are high in calories and packed with saturated fats. Changes in livestock feeding have also caused the CLA content in food to decline by nearly 80 per cent in the last two decades. You can make up for this shortfall by taking CLA supplements. Three 600–1,200 mg capsules should be taken daily before meals.

Co-enzyme Q10

helps with

- ❈ fainting and/or dizziness
- ❈ fatigue
- ❈ obesity

Co-Q10 is an important nutrient within the body's energy production process. Because Co-Q10 facilitates the production of energy, it may help burn calories which are normally converted to fat. One study showed that people on a low fat diet doubled their weight loss when they supplemented with Co-Q10.[9] Co-Q10 has also been proven useful in controlling blood sugar.

Co-Q10 is, however, best known as a heart-healthy supplement. One study published in the *American Journal of Cardiology* shows that heart patients taking Co-Q10 either alone or with other drugs lived an average of three years longer than those not taking Co-Q10. Co-Q10 can also lower blood pressure, which can reduce the risk of having a heart attack or stroke. It is routinely given to heart patients in Japan.

The usual dose is two 60 mg capsules twice a day. Ideally it should be taken under the guidance of a nutritional therapist.

Vitamin C

helps with

✿ acne
✿ diabetes
✿ excess hair
✿ fainting and/or dizziness
✿ fatigue
✿ hair loss
✿ insulin resistance
✿ irregular or absent periods
✿ mood swings
✿ obesity
✿ sleep problems/insomnia

A shortage of vitamin C, even if mild, can promote a wide range of illnesses and diseases, since vitamin C is a vital nutrient for the immune system. Research studies have shown that vitamin C helps with the clearance of toxic chemicals form the body, improves blood-sugar control, lowers blood cholesterol and generally promotes a feeling of health and well-being. It also speeds up a slow metabolism, promoting it to burn more calories, aids in improving scalp circulation, and some women find vitamin C creams useful for acne. It is an important nutrient for all women, and especially important for women with symptoms of PCOS such as insulin resistance, excess weight, acne, thinning hair and irregular periods.

The amount of vitamin C you need to ease PCOS symptoms and boost your health will not fit into a multivitamin and mineral. Supplementation should provide 1,000 mg of vitamin C, with at least 25 mg of bioflavonoids or other synergistic factors such as rosehips or berry extracts.

Damiana

helps with

* ✸ depression
* ✸ fainting and/or dizziness
* ✸ fatigue
* ✸ hot flushes/flashes
* ✸ irregular or absent periods
* ✸ mental fogginess
* ✸ mood swings

Regarded as an aphrodisiac in Central America, damiana is used by both men and women to maintain sexual health. Because of its balancing effect on hormones, damiana is often prescribed by homoeopaths to treat PCOS symptoms. Damiana also has a mildly stimulating property which enhances feelings of alertness and energy. Typical doses would be one 60 mg capsule three times a day.

Caution
Do not use if you are pregnant or trying to conceive.

Dandelion

helps with

* ✸ acne
* ✸ diabetes
* ✸ eating disorders
* ✸ fainting and/or dizziness
* ✸ fatigue
* ✸ irritability
* ✸ obesity
* ✸ water retention

Dandelion is used in virtually every tradition in the world as a herb to benefit the digestive system. It is among the most nutritionally-rich medicinal herbs, improving the function of the stomach and cleansing the liver. Both root and leaf can be used, or the juice extracted from the fresh plant. The root acts as a gentle liver-cleansing tonic, while the roasted root can be used in tea form for its diuretic qualities.

Dong Quai

helps with

❋ anaemia
❋ fainting and/or dizziness
❋ fatigue
❋ hot flushes/flashes
❋ infertility
❋ irregular or absent periods
❋ mood swings
❋ PMS symptoms

Dong quai is a Chinese herb (*Angelica*) made from the root of a large plant in the celery family. It is available in several forms, including capsules and liquid extracts. A two-month trial is suggested to determine effectiveness.

In Traditional Chinese Medicine dong quai is well known as a tonic for the female reproductive system, regulating hormonal control and improving the rhythm of the menstrual cycle. Dong quai is sometimes called the 'female ginseng' and is the most widely-used herb among Chinese women because of its reputation as a sex-enhancer, stress-beater and energy-enhancer.

The only known side-effect of dong quai is occasional sun sensitivity which may cause a rash. It is not recommended during menstruation or if any kind of blood problem is prevalent, as it promotes bleeding. Pregnant or breastfeeding women are not advised to use this herb.

Essential Fatty Acids

helps with

- ✿ acne (Omega-3)
- ✿ appetite control
- ✿ breast tenderness (Omega-3)
- ✿ depression (Omega-3)
- ✿ diabetes
- ✿ eating disorders (Omega-3)
- ✿ fainting and/or dizziness (Omega-3)
- ✿ fatigue (Omega-3)
- ✿ food cravings (Omega-3)
- ✿ hair loss (Omega-3)
- ✿ heart health
- ✿ hormonal balance
- ✿ infertility (Omega-3)
- ✿ insulin resistance (Omega-3)
- ✿ irregular or absent periods (Omega-3)
- ✿ irritability (Omega-3)
- ✿ mood swings (Omega-3)
- ✿ obesity
- ✿ skin and hair problems
- ✿ water retention (Omega-3)

Essential fatty acids, as we saw in Chapter 2, are crucial for healthy hormonal function and are needed by every cell in the body. They keep skin smooth and soft, repair damaged skin cells and dissolve fatty deposits that block pores. According to a recent animal study by Margaret T Behme MD of University Hospital London, Ontario, Omega-3 fatty acids, or fish oils, improve insulin sensitivity and reduce insulin resistance.[10] They help keep cell membranes flexible. Flexible cell membranes have more and more insulin receptors, which improves glucose metabolism.

On top of all this, another recent study linked a diet low in Omega-3 fatty acids to a higher incidence of depression. This is not surprising when you consider that the human brain consists of more than 50 per cent fat cells. Given that fatty acids play such a vital role in our health, many researchers believe that deficiency in essential fatty acids, especially Omega-3, is a leading cause of cancer and heart disease.

To meet your essential fat requirement, consume 1 or 2 tablespoons of a cold-pressed organic blend of seed oils providing Omega-3. The other possibility is to supplement with capsules. For Omega-3 this means flax seed oil or hempseed oil capsules, or the more concentrated fish oil capsules. High-strength fish oil is preferred as it contains the readily usable form.

As these essential fatty acids are so vital it is advisable, says Dr Marilyn Glenville, 'to supplement them in your diet in their most readily available form. Whatever supplement you choose, read the label on the back of the container and aim for a supplement that gives you at least 150 mg of GLA (Omega-6) per day. With EPA (Omega-3), aim for a supplement that will give you at least 2 g per day.'

If you are a vegetarian and prefer not to take fish oil, linseed oil contains both Omega-3 and Omega-6 EFAs. Take 15 ml (or g) per day of oil.

Evening Primrose Oil

helps with

❄ breast tenderness

Evening primrose oil, a Native American traditional remedy, is used by some women with PCOS to ease breast tenderness, water retention and mood swings. According to medical herbalist Ann Walker who treats many women with PCOS:

Breast pain is perhaps the only indication for evening primrose oil for women with PCOS, although it is also well known for improving the skin. It is high in Omega-6, which can exacerbate the problem. I would not use it in

PCOS. *Aim for 2 g of Omega-3 from fish oil (DHA and EPA) per day. Read the label to get this.*

Evening primrose oil is prescribed in the UK under the brand name Efamast. The dose recommended by doctors is around 1,000 mg per day.

Vitamin E

helps with

* ✽ diabetes
* ✽ hair loss
* ✽ infertility
* ✽ insulin resistance
* ✽ irregular or absent periods

Vitamin E is a powerful antioxidant. Like selenium, it plays a protective role in the body. Studies show that adding antioxidants such as vitamin C and vitamin E to an animal's diet significantly reduces age-related ovulation problems.[11] If you have PCOS and are over 35 and having problems conceiving, vitamin E in your diet could be of significant help. As well as boosting your immune system, balancing blood sugar, improving hair and skin condition, this important vitamin may also play a role in reducing the risk of heart disease, which is important news for women with PCOS who are insulin resistant.

We don't know the optimal level of vitamin E on a long-term basis, but evidence suggests that the best health effects of protective nutrients comes from the food we eat. Try to get an adequate supply of vitamin E from food sources such as nuts and nut butters from vegetable oils, especially sunflower and wheat germ oil, and ensure that any multivitamin and mineral you take contains 30 mg of vitamin E.

You want to get the most from your supplement so you should choose the natural version, known as d-alpha-tocopherol, and avoid the synthetic one which is called dl-alpha-tocopherol.
Dr Marilyn Glenville

A study in the *American Journal of Clinical Nutrition* has shown that natural vitamin E is absorbed better and works more efficiently than the synthetic version.

Fenugreek

helps with

❈ diabetes
❈ insulin resistance
❈ obesity

Fenugreek appears to lower blood-sugar levels by interfering with the digestion and absorption of sugars and improving the utilization of sugar once it is absorbed. Two studies published in the *European Journal of Clinical Nutrition* reported that fenugreek improves glucose intolerance in people with Type II diabetes by slowing down the rate of glucose absorption from the digestive tract.[12]

A dose of 25 to 50 mg of fenugreek seed powder twice daily with meals appears to be effective.

Caution
Fenugreek should not be used during pregnancy.

Flax Seed

helps with

❈ breast tenderness
❈ hair loss
❈ hair and skin problems
❈ insulin resistance
❈ irregular periods
❈ raised cholesterol levels
❈ sluggish metabolism

Flax seed (also known as linseed) is unique because it contains both of the essential fatty acids: Omega-3 and Omega-6. More importantly, it is the richest vegetarian source of the hard-to-get Omega-3 essential fatty acid. These healthy fats are necessary in aiding weight reduction because they help you metabolize fat better, lowering cholesterol, enhancing immunity and even nourishing the reproductive organs, skin, hair and bone tissue.

Up to six 1-gram capsules a day may be helpful. Flax oil, which is a food, can be taken by the spoonful: 1 tablespoon per day (15 grams) is commonly recommended, if you cannot take fish oil. Because of the strong taste you may prefer to take flax seed capsules.

Popular vegetable oils such as olive, sunflower, almond, avocado, sesame, peanut and corn, while containing varying amounts of Omega-6, contain negligible amounts of Omega-3. Of the readily available vegetable oils, only three contain both Omega-3 and Omega-6: flaxseed oil, hempseed oil, and soy oil. Since Omega-3 is low or even non-existent in the typical modern diet, flaxseed is by far the most desirable vegetable oil.

Garlic

helps with

❈ insulin resistance

Garlic may have a mild blood sugar-lowering effect. And, like oily fish and oats, garlic is also linked with heart health because it contains a substance which can stimulate your body to produce HDL (the good cholesterol).

Optimal doses are not known, but – taking your social life into account – try to consume reasonable amounts on a regular basis. You might want to grate it onto your food or take a one-a-day supplement.

Garcinia Cambogia

helps with

❋ insulin resistance
❋ weight loss

'If you find you are really struggling with sugar cravings, or you find it difficult to resist bingeing on just about anything, this is the supplement for you' says Dr Marilyn Glenville. *Garcinia cambogia* is a small tropical fruit than comes from central Asia. It contains hydroxy-citric-acid (HCA), which helps carbohydrates convert into energy instead of fat. The HCA seems to curb the appetite, reduce food intake and inhibit the formation of fat and cholesterol.

HCA is thought to help tune up the body's glucose and insulin metabolism. Animals fed a high HCA-supplemented diet have shown reduced food intake and a decline in body fat.

Some women with PCOS say that they don't eat so much and lose a lot of weight when taking HCA, though others see no positive effects. To be of maximum effect it needs to be incorporated into a sensible diet and exercise programme. Work with your doctor or natural health practitioner when taking weight-loss supplements of any kind.

Caution
This supplement must not be taken by pregnant or breastfeeding women.

Gingko Biloba

helps with

❋ mental fogginess

Gingko biloba has been shown to improve short-term memory and increase blood flow to the brain, which can encourage clearer thinking.

Experts agree that anyone with a circulatory problem – or at risk of developing one, as women with PCOS are – should take gingko biloba. Take up to three 60 mg capsules a day. Capsules need to be taken for at least two weeks to see results.

Gymnema Sylvestre

helps with

❊ diabetes
❊ insulin resistance

Native to India, this herb has been used by Indian healers for nearly 2,000 years, as part of the Ayurvedic traditional system of medicine, as a treatment for diabetes. Published studies show that it not only lowers blood-sugar levels but may help repair damaged cells in the pancreas, the gland in which insulin is produced, thereby improving insulin resistance. Although not scientifically proven, gymnema is reputed to reduce the urge to eat sweets and may be helpful for women with PCOS who experience food cravings and want to lose weight.

If you are taking medication for diabetes talk to your doctor before using gymnema.

Gymnema sylvestre is available in capsules. Take two 200 mg capsules a day. Gymnema extract (5–10 drops) can be mixed with tea, water or juice. Drink one cup daily.

Horsetail

helps with

❊ hair loss

Natural health practitioners have long recommended horsetail, a herb rich in the mineral silicon, to help restore dull, lifeless, thinning hair.

Although there is no scientific evidence to back this claim, some natural health practitioners prescribe silicon to forestall hair loss. Silicon levels decrease with age, and some researchers believe the decline in this mineral may cause connective tissue problems as well as wrinkles.

Take up to three 500 mg capsules or tablets up to three times a day.

Iron

helps with

✻ cracks at the side of the mouth
✻ fainting and/or dizziness
✻ fatigue
✻ hair loss
✻ infertility
✻ irregular or absent periods
✻ pale complexion
✻ sore tongue

You should only take iron if you know you have a deficiency. Your doctor can test you for this and advise on the correct supplement and dose to take. Heavy periods can cause iron deficiency, but iron deficiency can also cause heavy periods. Good food sources of iron include fish, poultry, leafy green vegetables and dried fruit. Apart from eating iron-rich foods you can increase your iron intake by not drinking tea with food. This is because the tannin contained in tea can block the uptake of iron and other minerals. Leave about an hour between eating and drinking tea. Cooking food in iron cookware or stainless steel, and avoiding the use of aluminium pans, can also increase your iron intake.

Iron deficiency should always be checked when there is an infertility problem, as taking iron is known to help women regain fertility. Iron supplements together with vitamin C have helped a number of women regain their fertility.[13]

Kelp

helps with

- ❀ acne
- ❀ hormonal imbalance
- ❀ irregular or absent periods
- ❀ obesity
- ❀ thyroid health

Kelp is thought to be useful in cases of obesity connected with thyroid deficiency. It contains iodine, the basic substance of thyroid hormones, and can help regulate the function of the thyroid gland to restore hormonal balance. Although kelp tablets are especially useful when there is a thyroid problem, they contain a rich supply of nutrients which can relieve ovulation and skin problems and promote weight loss. Alternatively, you can incorporate small amounts of seaweed and sea vegetables into your diet a couple of times a week.

L-carnitine

helps with

- ❀ fainting and/or dizziness
- ❀ fatigue
- ❀ insulin resistance
- ❀ obesity

L-carnitine is a vitamin-like nutrient involved in energy production that is found in the heart, brain and skeletal muscles. This supplement promises to make you stronger, sleeker and healthier. The more carnitine is available, the faster fat is transported and the more fat is used for energy. Evidence is anecdotal, but many women with PCOS feel that the supplement does increase energy, helps them lose weight and makes a real difference to the way they feel.

Take up to three 250 to 500 mg capsules or tablets daily, half an hour before eating or two hours afterwards.

Lecithin Granules

helps with

- ❈ irregular or absent periods
- ❈ obesity

Lecithin is a substance which helps assimilate and transport essential fatty acids, and aids fat metabolism, cholesterol and hormone regulation, brain function and reproduction. It may be helpful to women with PCOS who have irregular periods and or want to lose weight. It is widely used by the food industry as an emulsifier in products such as mayonnaise. It is also available as a food supplement to promote weight loss, usually in granules and capsules. Good food sources of lecithin include liver, meats, fish, wheat, peanuts and soybeans.

Liquorice

helps with

- ❈ acne
- ❈ excess hair
- ❈ irregular or absent periods
- ❈ obesity

This plant contains hormonally-active compounds categorized as saponins. A Japanese study found that liquorice was of help to women with infrequent periods. The study also found that liquorice helped women with elevated testosterone and low oestrogen levels, which can often occur in women with PCOS. It is an adaptogen, and appears to strengthen oestrogen when levels fall too low, and inhibit oestrogen when levels climb too high. In addition, liquorice root has a real affinity with the liver and is thought to be a powerful detoxifier. It can also stimulate the adrenal gland and improve thyroid function.

Caution
This herb should only be taken under professional supervision. Do not use this herb for more than seven consecutive days, and avoid completely if you have high blood pressure, are pregnant, or have diabetes or severe menstrual problems.

Living Sprouts

helps with

❀ fainting and/or dizziness
❀ fatigue

Living sprouts are bursting with nutrients which can improve digestion, vitality and energy. One of the greatest studies ever conducted in the field of natural health was supervised by Dr Edmond Bordeaux Szekely over a period of 33 years, during which time he evaluated over 120,000 people on the experimental effects of eating raw foods.[14] In this study he identified the most life-enhancing, high-energy, nutrient-rich food as the biogenic category which consists of all sprouts.

Millet and quinoa sprouts are often thought to have the most therapeutic health benefits for mind and body. In addition to these grains, wheat, rye, oats, barley, seeds, nuts and pulses can also be sprouted.

Ideally, living sprouts should move from supplement status to form an important part of your daily diet. You can easily sprout seeds and beans at home. Try clover, alfalfa seeds, mung seeds, fenugreek and wheatberries, for example.

Magnesium

helps with

❀ diabetes
❀ fainting and/or dizziness

* ✸ fatigue
* ✸ hot flushes/flashes
* ✸ insulin resistance
* ✸ irritability
* ✸ mood swings
* ✸ sleep problems/insomnia

Magnesium strengthens bones and teeth, and promotes healthy muscles by helping them to relax. It is also essential for energy-production. It is used by the body at the very first stage of the process which converts glucose to energy. Magnesium deficiency has been linked to symptoms of PMS, diabetes, mood swings, muscle weakness, insomnia, mental confusion and depression. There is a strong link between magnesium deficiency and insulin resistance,[15] so it is important to include it if you have PCOS.

If you want to supplement with magnesium, amino acid chelate and citrate are twice as well absorbed as magnesium carbonate or oxide. You should not consume more than 600 mg of magnesium a day. Recommended daily intake is in the region of 300 mg.

Manganese

helps with

* ✸ diabetes
* ✸ infertility
* ✸ insulin resistance
* ✸ mood swings

Manganese is an essential trace element needed for healthy skin, bone and cartilage formation and to regulate blood-sugar levels. Deficiency is often found in those with diabetes. It can thus be helpful for women with diabetes and/or insulin resistance. Good food sources include wholemeal bread, nuts, pulses (beans), fruit, green leaf vegetables and cereals. There should be no need for supplementation if your diet is good. A cup of tea can provide up to half of the required daily intake (from 0.5 to 5.0 mg).

Milk Thistle

helps with

- ❋ acne
- ❋ eating disorders
- ❋ fainting and/or dizziness
- ❋ fatigue
- ❋ hot flushes/flashes
- ❋ irritability
- ❋ liver health

Since ancient times milk thistle has been the primary herb used to treat liver disorders. Modern research has confirmed that *Silymarin*, the collective name for the substances found in milk thistle which produce this beneficial effect, do indeed enhance liver function. A number of studies have shown that milk thistle can result in an increase of new liver cells to replace old, damaged ones.[16] Some naturopaths recommend milk thistle to anyone who is taking any kind of medication, to help keep liver enzymes normal. Don't get the idea, though, that milk thistle is used for people with specific liver disorders, where specialist treatment is always recommended.

Many natural therapists recommend up to three 500 mg tablets of capsules daily for women with PCOS, to help them gently detox. This potent liver protector is also helpful for symptoms of PMT, acne, stress and fatigue, and is an important preventative herb if you smoke, drink a lot of alcohol or live in a polluted area.

Motherwort

helps with

- ❋ breast tenderness
- ❋ hot flushes/flashes
- ❋ infertility

❋ irregular or absent periods
❋ irritability

Motherwort is thought to affect the nervous, cardiac and female reproductive systems. It is popular for treating anxiety, tension, nervous disorders and symptoms of PMS. Some women with PCOS find drinking motherwort tea helps reduce anxiety and PMS symptoms, and promotes relaxation.

Psyllium Husks

helps with

❋ food cravings
❋ insulin resistance
❋ obesity

Psyllium is a grain grown in India that is utilized for its fibre content. A good intestinal cleanser and stool softener, it is one of the most popular sources of fibre used by women with PCOS. It thickens very quickly when mixed with liquid and must be consumed quickly. The high fibre content makes it especially good for women with PCOS who have blood-sugar problems, reducing food cravings and cutting down hunger pangs.

Red Raspberry Leaf

helps with

❋ acne
❋ hot flushes/flashes
❋ infertility
❋ irregular or absent periods

Red raspberry leaf is a native European shrub that has been used by women for centuries as a herbal tonic, usually in tea form. It is non-toxic and can be taken safely every day, even during pregnancy.

Red raspberry leaf contains a high concentration of vitamins and minerals. Chemical analyses report that the herb contains oestrogen-like compounds which promote fertility. It also decreases heavy menstrual bleeding and strengthens the uterus. An added benefit is that it can alleviate mild diarrhoea.

St John's Wort

helps with

❄ mild to moderate depression

St John's Wort (*Hypericum perforatum*), the herb billed as nature's Prozac, has the ability to work as an effective antidepressant. It is prescribed by German doctors more often than antidepressant drugs. A recent overview of 23 clinical trials into St John's Wort and depression was carried out by Klaus Linde and colleagues and published in the *British Medical Journal*, declaring Hypericum to be superior to placebo and just as effective as antidepressant medication for mild to moderate depression.[17] Severe depression always needs medical attention.

Reported side-effects include mild nausea and skin rash but, unlike many antidepressant drugs, St John's Wort has not been found to lower sex drive.

There are many brands of St John's Wort on the market, and they can vary in strength and potency. The dose of 900 mg daily has been shown by studies to be effective in counteracting mild depression. However, over-the-counter preparations only provide 300 mg per day. Visiting a registered medical herbalist for a tailor-made prescription is one good way to make sure you are getting the correct dose.

In addition to St John's Wort, other herbs which are thought to relieve depression include ginger, gingko biloba, liquorice root, oat straw, peppermint, lemon balm and Siberian ginseng. A medical herbalist can help you choose what's best for you.

Caution

Take care with the use of St John's Wort if you are on the contraceptive pill. According to Dr Ann Walker,

> *It has not been proven that St John's Wort taken alongside the contraceptive pill results in a greater number of unwanted pregnancies. We do know that the detoxifying effect of this herb reduces blood levels of drugs and it is possible that this can reduce the level of contraceptive effectiveness in some women.*

Saw Palmetto

helps with

❋ acne
❋ excess hair

The herb's active ingredient is unknown, but European studies have shown that it seems to be able to counteract the effects of excess testosterone. Saw palmetto has been traditionally used against prostate troubles, and numerous studies have confirmed that it is effective in slowing down the conversion of testosterone. 'Add saw palmetto to your treatment plan,' says Dr Glenville 'if you have excess hair growth or have been told you have high levels of androgens.'

Shatawari

helps with

❋ diabetes
❋ irregular or absent periods

A member of the asparagus family, shatawari is a popular Ayurvedic tonic reputed to enhance a woman's sexual vitality. It is used by some women to help normalize the hormonal imbalances of PCOS. Take as prescribed by an experienced practitioner.

Siberian Ginseng

helps with

- ✿ depression
- ✿ diabetes
- ✿ fainting and/or dizziness
- ✿ fatigue
- ✿ infertility
- ✿ insulin resistance
- ✿ irregular or absent periods
- ✿ sleep problems/insomnia

Known as an adaptogenic herb (adapting itself to your individual needs), Siberian ginseng is believed to help the body adapt to stress, including the metabolic stress of fluctuating blood glucose levels. It is frequently recommended to women with PCOS and has few side-effects.

Ginseng is currently under investigation as a possible future replacement for insulin in diabetics. Research from Canada has found that ginseng taken before or after eating reduces blood-sugar levels. A 20 per cent reduction in blood-sugar levels was recorded when ginseng was eaten after a meal. Siberian ginseng aids in moving fluids and nutrients around the body, and reduces the stress of adjusting to a new diet.

Generally it's best to take ginseng in the morning, since some women have trouble sleeping if they take it later in the day. According to research in Germany, ginseng can, on rare occasions, raise blood pressure, so it's a good idea to have your blood pressure monitored first, as women with PCOS have an increased risk of blood pressure problems. A typical daily dose is 100 to 200 mg of a standardized ginseng product.

Soy Concentrate (Isolates)

helps with

❋ breast tenderness
❋ hot flushes/flashes
❋ irregular or absent periods
❋ irritability

Phytoestrogens are substances that occur naturally in foods; they can have a balancing effect on your hormones.[18] One study showed that eating soya increased oestrogen effectiveness when levels were low, and reduced its effectiveness when they were high. This explains why soya beans can reduce hot flushes for women going through menopause (when it is thought there is an oestrogen deficiency) and reduce the incidence of breast cancer (often due to excess oestrogen).

Soy products and tofu are both excellent sources of isoflavones, which are powerful phytoestrogens. Rich in the isoflavones genistein and daidzein, soy products may also protect against breast cancer and heart disease.[19]

In one Australian study, 58 menopausal women who had at least 214 hot flushes a week were given 45 g of soy flour daily in the form of baked goods. Within a six-week period, these women reported a 40 per cent decline in symptoms. Research has also shown that phytoestrogens can help to produce lighter periods and to lengthen the cycle in women whose cycles are too short.[20]

A whole range of soy supplements are now readily available in health food stores. Sprouted soy concentrate is a particularly potent source of these important phytoestrogens. Take two tablets a day. Be sure the soy supplements contain genistein and daidzein (the usual dose is 50 mg of genistein and daidzein, along with other isoflavones).

If you are thinking about supplementing with soy, check with your doctor first and take the supplement in moderation. Soya can be good for you, but it is not meant to be eaten in excessive quantities. If possible get your phytoestrogens from the food you eat rather than a supplement.

Supplements never offer the same beneficial effects that foods can. My recommendation is to use soya supplements in the short term to help combat symptoms. At the same time, however you should also make changes in your diet and start to include phytoestrogens in your cooking.
Dr Marilyn Glenville

Try to eat your soy products in their traditional form, such as miso, soy or organic soya milks, and avoid gimmicky soya bars and snacks unless they are made from whole beans. Variety is the key to a healthy diet, so don't forget that soya is just one of many phytoestrogens. Phytoestrogens are found in other legumes such as lentils and chickpeas, most fruits and vegetables, wheat, alfalfa, hops, fennel, celery and rhubarb, and the herbs sage, fennel and parsley.

Spirulina

helps with

- ❋ acne
- ❋ depression
- ❋ fainting and/or dizziness
- ❋ fatigue
- ❋ food cravings
- ❋ insulin resistance
- ❋ obesity

Spirulina is an algae and a concentrated source of high quality, easily digestible nutrients especially beneficial for women with PCOS. It is available from most health food shops. It stimulates the discharge of toxic residues in the body, calms blood sugar and keeps your appetite under control. Take 4 spirulina tablets a day, or add 4 tablespoons of powder to a smoothie in your blender.

Triphala

helps with

❋ obesity

Triphala, a combination of dried fruits from several plants is the most widely used herbal preparation in Ayurvedic medicine. It can be taken alone or in combination with other herbs. In particular triphala is reputed to normalize digestion, enhance nutrient absorption and regulate metabolism. In one recent Indian study, triphala was successfully used to promote weight loss.

Turmeric

helps with

❋ diabetes
❋ insulin resistance

Ayurvedic doctors view turmeric as an effective treatment for controlling high blood sugar. It is also thought to be able to strengthen digestion, decongest the liver and improve flexibility by softening tight muscles and joints. Ask a practitioner about taking turmeric capsules before meals for a month, then have your condition re-evaluated. Another way to take turmeric is to mix half a teaspoon of the spice with half a teaspoon of ground bay leaf mixed in with 1 tablespoon of aloe vera juice. Take twice a day before lunch and dinner.

Other Ayurvedic herbs believed to boost insulin production include bitter melon, tulsi or sacred basil, and gymnema sylvestre.

Unicorn Root

helps with

❀ infertility
❀ irregular or absent periods

A uterine tonic, unicorn root, also called blazing star, is a North American herb said to be useful for women who have delayed or absent periods. This herb may also help prevent miscarriage and menstrual bleeding due to uterine weakness. It is often found in women's herbal compounds as it has a balancing effect on hormones. 'Mixed with other herbs it can be given for ovarian cysts or endometriosis,' says Dr Glenville. However, this herb is an endangered species, so is used only sparingly by herbalists. Another herb which, like Unicorn root, helps to normalize the balance of hormones is White Peony.

Unkei-to

helps with

❀ irregular or absent periods

This Japanese herbal mixture may help to encourage ovulation in women with PCOS. Unkei-to is a blend of 12 herbs including ginseng, evodia fruit and ginger stem. Scientists at Osaka Medical College in Japan gave 52 women 7.5 g a day of unkei-to for four weeks, and 48 controls no treatment. The researchers found that over half the women who took the herbal combination reported successful ovulation and an improvement in their menstrual cycle. No studies have been conducted into the effectiveness of unkei-to for women with PCOS, but if you have irregular periods it may be beneficial if taken under the guidance of a doctor.

Valerian

helps with

❋ sleep problems/insomnia

Valerian is a herbal sedative which can help you get a good night's sleep without the hangover effect of traditional sleeping pills. Hops and passiflora may also help with sleep problems.

Vanadium

helps with

❋ insulin resistance

The mineral vanadium, found in vanadyl sulphate supplements, helps improve insulin's ability to transport glucose into cells. With insulin working efficiently, the body needs and produces less of it. According to Barbara F Harland, PhD, of Howard University, Washington DC, vanadium has been researched for 40 years and is close to being recognized as an essential nutrient for people with diabetes.[21]

Vanadium has been used by doctors and natural therapists as part of the treatment for women with PCOS and insulin resistance or diabetes. It is not normally available as a supplement, but foods rich in vanadium include parsley, lobster, radishes, lettuce, bonemeal and gelatin.

Wild Yam

helps with

❋ hot flushes/flashes
❋ infertility
❋ irregular or absent periods
❋ irritability

In its crude form, wild yam is an anti-inflammatory agent with a weak hormonal activity in the body which may improve fertility. It has a progesterone-favourable effect in the body. Wild Yam is rich in disgenin, from which progestin is made in the lab, but the creams sold as 'wild yam' are not the same as progesterone creams and do not have the same measurable effects. Although the progesterone in these creams is derived from Wild Yam, it has undergone chemical modification.

Wild yam is used in tincture form, as topical creams and gels, in capsules, teas and tablets, and sublingually (under the tongue). It has therapeutic value in preventing miscarriage, but women with PCOS may find it helpful for the treatment of PMS, uterine cramps, abdominal colic and menstrual irregularity.

Zinc

helps with

* ❀ acne
* ❀ eating disorders
* ❀ fainting and/or dizziness
* ❀ fatigue
* ❀ infertility
* ❀ insulin resistance
* ❀ mood swings
* ❀ obesity

Zinc plays an important role in the synthesis, storage and secretion of insulin, and is therefore important for women with PCOS and insulin resistance. It is water soluble and can be lost when urination increases. Low levels of zinc affect the ability of the pancreas to produce and secrete insulin.

Zinc works as an antioxidant by protecting the body's cells from free radical damage. If zinc levels are low, your immune system will not function properly because it needs zinc to fight off viruses and bacteria, and there could be problems with fertility as zinc is necessary for a healthy reproductive cycle. You may also become more vulnerable to depression.

Zinc has also been advocated in the treatment of eating disorders. Finally, zinc is excellent for problem skin. It helps reduce the inflammation response within the body and aids healing.

The body is more efficient at absorbing zinc from foods such as beans and other pulses, shellfish and fish, wholegrain foods, nuts and dairy foods, than from tablets. Manufacturers often add zinc to breakfast cereals; you may get your zinc this way. Nevertheless, much of the zinc could have been lost in food processing, so to boost your zinc intake eat more wholegrains and make sure your multivitamin and mineral contains zinc.

If you don't think you are getting enough zinc you may want to take a daily 15 mg supplement – don't take any more than this, though, as high zinc levels may make you vulnerable to bacterial and viral infections.

My periods were regular until I was 19. Then they stopped, and in 10 months I put on 20 lb and got very depressed and frustrated because I couldn't understand why I was putting on weight when I had never been fat before and my diet hadn't changed. I also felt very unfeminine and noticed that I was getting hairier. I went to my doctor, who told me that if I lost weight I would feel better. He made me feel worse because he just assumed I was lazy about my weight/appearance.

I went to a library and borrowed a book on herbs. I began taking a good multivitamin and mineral supplement, and agnus castus along with other 'female toner' teas. After 8 months I got my periods back, but they were irregular. I also started to lose weight. Then I got a massive, painful, heavy bleed which lasted five weeks. I found a different doctor, who listened to me and ordered some tests which confirmed PCOS. I decided not to go on the Pill or take medication. Instead I visited a medical herbalist for a personalized pack of herbal supplements, and started to read up about blood-sugar problems and how they can be managed through diet.

So far, so good. I've had normal regular periods for a year and my weight is steady. I still get facial hair, which gets me down. I get tired of plucking, shaving and waxing, especially my face. It makes me feel angry and cheated, and sometimes I want to hide from the world for ever. But I am thankful that so far I am managing my other symptoms OK, and perhaps one day I'll find an answer for my hirsutism. I just want everyone out there who feels like me about their PCOS to hold their head up, stop feeling they are helpless – there are positive things we can do to improve our health – be strong and remember we're all beautiful in our own special ways.
Alira, 21

Part Three

PREPARE FOR SUCCESS:

MOTIVATION, SUPPORT AND A
HEALTHY ATTITUDE TO FOOD

9

Getting Motivated for Change

So, you've read this far and now want to make a change – but how do you fit change into your busy life?

In an ideal world, we would all make healthy food choices and get plenty of time for exercise and relaxation. But this is the real world, and it can often be hard to kick old habits and create change.

I know I need to start eating better. Last year I went on holiday in Greece and we ate masses of fruits and vegetables and other healthy stuff. I felt terrific. I lost weight, my acne cleared and I didn't get PMS. I tried hard to keep it up when I got back, but I work long hours. There is always mountains of housework to do, and any free time I get I spend with my mother, who is getting very frail and needs a lot of looking after. I don't even have time to get enough sleep, how am I going to find time to think about my diet?
Mary, 40

Perhaps your job is stressful and it doesn't allow you time to think about your diet. Perhaps your partner likes you to join him or her in heavy late-night suppers. Perhaps your children are so demanding you haven't got any energy left to take care of yourself. If there are certain things in your life which are preventing or making it difficult for you to change the way you eat, you need to have a good long think about whether or not you have your priorities right.

Is your job really so demanding that you can't make healthy food choices? Is your partner so selfish that he or she expects you to eat unhealthy foods and jeopardize your health? Yes, children and looking after ill relatives can be exhausting, but the healthier you are, the better you will be able to cope. If your mum insists that you eat the wrong kinds of foods, explain to her that you are concerned about your health and need to make changes.

Nothing is more important than your health. Once you, and those around you, realize that your health is your first priority, you'll discover that there is always room for positive change in your life which can fit around your existing commitments and relationships.

THE ART OF HEALTHY EATING

Once you've decided you are prepared to make changes, the process of healthy eating begins in earnest. You have read this book and discovered how to eat to help alleviate your PCOS symptoms. The challenge for you now is:

- getting motivated
- changing old habits
- sticking to your new eating plan long enough to see some benefits, and staying with it even once you start to feel better.

Dietary change, as any dietician will tell you, is not simply based on the food you eat. It's also based on how, when, where, what and why you eat.

The first step is to *change your attitude towards food*.

What does this mean, exactly?

It means that if you are trying to change your eating habits you must *want* to change your eating habits. More importantly, you must want to eat healthily for *yourself*, not for others.

Change Your Mind

My mother, my sister, my nana were always telling me to eat properly and lose weight. Then my doctor told me that I had PCOS and I needed to watch my weight. I've lost count of the times I've started a diet, lost a few pounds and then put them all back on again. It wasn't until I decided I wanted to become an air hostess that I actually lost weight and kept it off. You see, I had to be considered healthy and fit to fly.
Amy, 23

The motivation to change your lifestyle has to come from within. It's like stopping smoking. No one else can make you do it. Attitude is everything. Study after study has shown that when a challenge presents itself, your success rate rises or falls on your degree of commitment. So give yourself short-term goals – such as getting into a dress a size smaller or seeking advice to improve/treat acne. Bear in mind that everyone will have different goals, and what your friend may consider important may be the thing that matters least to you. It's what *you* think and feel that matter the most here.

To get the job done, it is important that you change your diet because *you* want to, not because your doctor has advised it or your loved ones urge it. Where does this conviction come from?

1 A desire to improve and maintain your health and specifically to control your symptoms, prevent the possibility of diabetes and heart disease and maximize your chances of health and a long life.
2 A desire to lose weight, if you have weight to lose, and feel your physical best.
3 A desire to feel good mentally – to be more confident, have more self-esteem and experience all-round feelings of accomplishment, fulfilment and satisfaction.

Three excellent reasons, and three powerful motivators: better health, improved body image, and an increased sense of mental and emotional well-being. If you can keep these three reasons in mind while you start to change your diet, your path will be much easier.

The very fact that you have got this far in reading this book shows that you are motivated to make changes. In fact, women with PCOS tend to be highly motivated, according to dietitians Sally Wharmby and Claire Mellors. 'In our experience they really want to make changes. Weight-reduction isn't their only goal, either. Good health and control of symptoms is, too.'

There are some simple strategies you can put in place to prepare yourself for success in following the healthy eating plan outlined in this book.

IDENTIFY YOUR TRIGGERS

I always reach for snacks, crisps and chocolate, all the kinds of food my doctor wants me to avoid, when I'm by myself. I guess I'm not very good at being alone.
Charlotte, 19

I'm usually very good during the day. I make healthy food choices, but in the evening that all goes out the window. The day is over and I find myself constantly eating. I'm not sure why.
Mandy, 26

If I know there is ice-cream in the fridge I have to eat it. If the kids don't eat all their food, I'll finish it for them. I'm the same at work. If someone brings in a box of chocolates or there is a birthday cake to share, I can't resist.
Laura, 45

In order to make change possible, you need to establish an environment that works for you by identifying the foods and situations that trigger unhealthy eating habits.

Sally Wharmby and Claire Mellors, Senior Dietitians at Queens Medical Centre, Nottingham, UK, who hold special PCOS nutrition and weight-loss clinics, stress the importance of looking at your specific circumstances to see where changes can be fitted into your life, and identifying obstacles and barriers. 'We urge you to keep a diary to identify areas to trouble-shoot. For instance, you may think you are eating regularly, but a diary may reveal snacking habits at work. If you have kids you may not realize how much of their food you are eating. A diary can really help you identify problem areas and negotiate changes that need to be made.'

Write down everything you eat and drink each day, noting how you feel before and after eating or drinking. It's better to write soon after you have eaten, rather than leaving things to the end of the day when you may not remember exact details. Be as honest as you can. Biscuit crumbs and leftovers have calories too! Sometimes becoming more aware of what you actually *do* eat, and not what you *think* you eat, can help you see where changes need to be made.

Do you always have a full biscuit tin? Do you have full-fat milk in the fridge? Is there a chocolate drawer in your house? Work out which practical temptations trigger your hunger for foods which aren't going to help you. Then eliminate them from the table, shelf and fridge. That's the first step.

Next, consider what time of day you are most likely to make unhealthy food choices. Mid-morning? Mid-afternoon? Midnight? Have a stock of healthy alternatives on hand.

And don't forget social eating. If you tend to eat high-calorie, high-fat foods at restaurants, choose restaurants that offer healthier options. If family meals are a problem, talk to your family and explain why you need to eat healthily. Get another family member to help you monitor what you eat. Pay attention to these and similar cues, and you'll find that you've done part of the work simply by acknowledging and coping with the situation.

GIVE UP NEGATIVE SELF-BELIEF

Personal trainers Pete Cohen and Judith Verity run a UK nationwide weight-loss and healthy eating group called Lighten Up. All that Lighten Up requires you to do is give up negative self-belief. After mastering this, you learn to eat when you're hungry, stop when you're full, choose the foods you need and find the motivation to get active.

Below are some motivational mindset-changing exercises recommended by Lighten Up for women with PCOS which can be particularly helpful if you are starting (or need motivation to continue) a healthy eating programme. (You can find more details of the Lighten Up healthy eating and weight-management system in Chapter 12.)

1) 'I'm Starting!'

Old habits really do die hard and change of any kind is always stressful. A good way to get started on any major life change is to conjure up powerful images of how you will look and feel if things *don't* change in your life. Perhaps poor health and weight gain limit your movements? Do you feel constantly tired and low?

Sometimes you need a reminder of what might happen if you don't take care of yourself. The technique also helps you focus on the real reasons why you want to change your eating habits. Think about how improved health and weight loss, if you need it, will improve your health, your relationships and your self-esteem now and in the years to come.

2) 'I'm Slipping!'

In order to keep going once you've made a start, try picturing yourself as you will be if you stick with it. Your hair is shiny, your skin soft and smooth, your periods are regular. You are slimmer, healthier, fitter, and feel fully in control of your life and able to cope with your problems.

You then can link this vision with healthy eating or exercise sessions. See yourself eating healthy food and enjoying it. See yourself having lots of energy to exercise. This isn't something you do once. You need to do it over and over again until it becomes a habitual way of thinking, on a daily basis.

3) 'It Takes Such a Long Time!'

You can help yourself stay patient and positive with daily motivational statements, night and morning, such as:

> 'I can manage my PCOS.'
> 'I'm slimmer, fitter and healthier.'
> 'I'm looking and feeling good.'
> 'The quality of my life is improving every day.'

Affirmations won't make you slimmer or healthier, but they can help you on your way to health and happiness. They give you that 'oomph' factor, that boost you need to keep going.

You can also help your motivation levels with a diary. At the end of each week, ask yourself these three questions:

1 Do I feel good?
2 Do I have lots of energy?
3 Am I enjoying my food and my exercise routine?

If the answer to any of the above is 'no', it's probable that you are pushing yourself too hard. It's time to change your routine and work towards more achievable exercise and healthy eating goals.

4) 'I Feel Great and Want to Stay that Way'

When you have a really good feeling about yourself and the changes you are making, acknowledge that feeling and dwell on it. If you have two regular periods in a row, for instance, or you just feel fitter and slimmer, make sure you make a mental note. We all have a tendency to dwell on the bad feelings, and even seek them out. When you are feeling good or pleased with your progress, give yourself another of those pats on the back, or even treat yourself to a walk in your favourite park, a favourite movie, a day off with your partner or a phone call to a treasured friend, and remember that feeling. Spend some time daydreaming, playing a film in your mind in which you are looking good and living a healthy life. Watch that film over and over again, whenever you need a boost.

10

Set Yourself Up for Success

Having read the PCOS diet guidelines in Chapters 2 and 3, you will recognize where changes in your eating habits need to be made. It's important to understand where you need to change, but remember to *take your time*. It's very difficult to change everything at once. Don't set yourself up to fail. Even if you are the kind of person who can cope with multiple changes, remember that those around you, including family and friends, may not be able to.

Start slowly and gradually. Healthy eating isn't about a short-term fix, it's about re-educating all your eating habits for life. Small and gradual changes are the best way to create long-term improvements in your health and well-being. These dietary changes are designed to get right to the heart of the underlying hormonal imbalances that cause PCOS, rather than simply treating the symptoms that appear as a result of them.

ONE SMALL STEP ...

In addition to working on a more positive mindset, you also need to take things one step at a time. As far as healthy eating and weight loss are concerned, patience is a virtue. It may have taken many years to get to the position you are in at the moment, so it is likely to take some time to reverse it.

To be successful, give yourself and those you live with some time. This does not mean you should do nothing. You are not going on a fad diet. You are gradually changing the way you (and possibly those around you) live.

'This is a big hurdle for many of the women we treat with PCOS,' say Sally and Claire. 'We try to explain why PCOS can't be treated with quick-fix diets. Although it seems the odds are against you because of your condition, you can lose weight and feel healthy if you make simple and gradual changes. Focus on simple steps, like establishing regular meals so that you have regular packets of energy throughout the day. Every small step is one step closer to feeling fitter, healthier and happier.'

Avoid, at all costs, quick-fix diets that promise immediate results. Find a nutritious alternative. Don't be taken in by claims made about the latest fad diets; they don't work for long-term health. If the claims seem too good to be true, they usually are. It is far better to follow a diet that suits your personal needs. (If you prefer following a specific plan, refer back to the chart in Chapter 2 for guidance on which ones can be useful.)

It typically takes about three months before you'll see major change. The full benefits may take many months or even years, although even after a week or two most people will notice considerable improvement. It can be difficult to stick to resolutions to change your eating habits if you don't see results immediately. But the advantage of taking things one day at a time is that you will tend to get long-lasting results. Think of it like saving – if you look after the small things today (the pennies, or in this case any day-to-day activities that could help you avoid getting acne, or having to move up into that next dress size), then the bigger things will look after themselves (the heart disease and the diabetes). So identify some small goals and you can start improving your life right now.

TIMING IS EVERYTHING

Start your new eating plan at the right time. If you are under a great deal of stress right now, if your life is in a period of flux, if there is a major change or crisis taking place, you don't need the pressure of a diet to complicate your life further. Wait until things settle down. Then, when your life is on an even keel again, go for it. Studies have shown that women who begin dieting in an untroubled state of mind tend to succeed more than those who are worried and depressed. But bear in mind that with PCOS you can feel down or low a lot of the time – you should try not to use this as an excuse NOT to start your plan. By all means, give yourself a break if you're going through an unexpected crisis or time of pressure, but be ready, too, to give yourself a motivational boost if you've got those 'everyday' PCOS blues – and you'll find that your new healthy lifestyle helps to get rid of them!

IT WON'T BE EASY

Changing my eating habits has been the hardest challenge I have ever faced. It took a lot of effort and will-power, and there were times when I felt I was making no progress, but, my goodness was it worth it. I feel like a new woman. My periods are regular, my acne has cleared and I'm expecting my first baby next year.
Amber, 33

There is no point pretending that change is easy – it isn't!

It takes a while before any change starts to feel comfortable or natural. But in the end you may find it hard to imagine that you could ever have enjoyed things that weren't good for you.

If you have ever tried to stop taking sugar in your tea or coffee, you will know that at first the drink tastes terrible, but soon you get to the stage where you think it tastes awful with the sugar back in. The same applies to drinking less coffee – the first few days you feel on edge and prone to headaches, but in time you find that caffeine has lost its appeal.

When you make changes they may not feel, taste, look, smell or even sound fun at the time, but if they're based on sound, sensible advice and you give yourself time to feel the benefits, you need never look back. You will start feeling healthier and happier and see a real improvement in the quality of your life.

BE GENTLE ON YOURSELF

Realize that you will inevitably experience periods when no matter how hard you try you can't lose weight or you slip back into old habits. When this happens, don't lose heart. It's all part of the healthy eating process. A good trick for getting past these times is to increase the amount that you exercise. Just know in advance that plateaux are bound to come. They happen to everyone. But know too that they will pass, and that they will be followed by periods of gratifying weight loss, if you have weight to lose, and a healthier you.

Now and then you will give in to those cravings for junk food, if you're human! Chances are you'll slip and slip again on the road to healthy eating. When you do, don't beat yourself up. Guilt and self-chastisement are pointless and demoralizing. Just tell yourself that tomorrow is another day. Then try again. When it comes to eating well, positive thinking and tackling things one day at a time take you a long way.

GET SUPPORT

The healthy eating guidelines in this book will give you general rules to allow you to plan and start to move in the right direction to achieve your personal goals. However, every one of us is unique, and what works for you may have different results for someone else. Where possible it's best to enlist the support of a healthcare team, your partner, if you have one, and your family, colleagues and friends.

Sally and Claire invite women with PCOS to bring partners, family and friends with them to consultations. 'We believe that explaining to loved ones why healthy eating is so crucial if you have PCOS, can try to encourage the whole family to eat healthily too and to support you.'

I'm the main earner and my partner looks after our little girl and does all the cooking. It was hard because I had to tell him that a lot of the food he was serving us wasn't that good for me. It was making my symptoms worse. Thankfully he didn't take offence. He went out and bought a cookbook and we are all eating much more healthily. Not only do I feel better, but we all do. My little girl concentrates a lot more and my partner and I have both started running again.
Sarah, 38

Much, of course, depends on the kind of person you are. If you're the sociable type and feel that a problem shared is a problem halved, the support of others when you change your eating habits may be invaluable to you. If, on the other hand, you're the independent type who likes to do things your way, you might find the pressure of family, friends and groups unwelcome. Although you seem self-contained, you are probably quite sensitive and prefer to analyse your feelings and motivations alone. You are the best judge of what will help you most.

You can help yourself get through the bad days and celebrate good days by gathering together your own support network. This can come ready-made in the form of a self-help group, or it can be a web of people you talk to about PCOS. Besides partners, family, friends and healthcare workers, an excellent place to turn for support can be found in PCOS support groups such as Verity and PCOSupport, as well as e-groups on the internet (for more suggestions, see Chapter 12).

PCOS made me feel really different from everyone else, and for a while I felt too embarrassed to talk to anyone about it because I thought they wouldn't understand. Joining Verity was virtually a lifesaver for me, giving me the opportunity to meet other women with PCOS and exchange information.

I don't feel alone anymore. I'm part of a community of women who understand exactly what I am going through. That's very comforting.
Jane, 28

The people in your support network need to know how you are and what PCOS is, as well as how you feel about it, so that at times of high emotion when you may not be as coherent as you would like, they know what you mean and won't say anything that makes you feel worse just because they don't understand.

11

Healing Your Emotional Relationship with Food

How many women do you know who have never been on a diet? How many of your friends have never said, 'I'd better not' about having dessert? How many times have you avoided telling someone how much you weigh?

Most women don't have a totally normal, healthy relationship with food, regardless of whether they have PCOS or not. There are loads of reasons why our relationship with food can be complex, such as concern about weight, or eating in response to difficult and painful emotions, but with PCOS the importance of food- and weight-management, feelings of stress and frustration, and insecurities about body image can intensify the problem.

However, in order to be able to change to a healthy eating plan, you need to heal your emotional relationship with food, otherwise you are putting yourself under greater pressure and can be setting yourself up to fail – which will only make your relationship with food even more complicated in the long run.

Sometimes I feel so low that only a chocolate bar can cheer me up. I eat one and feel like I have let myself down, so I eat another one, followed by cakes, chips, sweets – anything I can lay my hands on. By the time I go to bed I feel tired, heavy, spotty and very, very guilty.
Monica, 32

I try to be positive, but it's very hard. I often cry, especially when I compare myself to 'normal' women my age. My sister, who has worse PCOS than me, says I am very lucky I don't have the terrible PCOS symptoms she has, no hairiness, bad skin or diabetes. I'm overweight but not obese. I battle to lose weight, but gain weight by just looking at food.
Nicole, 30

It was after my second miscarriage that my eating spiralled out of control. I didn't notice or care what I put into my mouth. I put on lots of weight. My periods stopped and my hair started to fall out, but it wasn't until my doctor told me that if I continued to put on weight I might not fall pregnant again that I started to become aware of how much damage I was doing to myself.
Lorinda, 34

COMFORT EATING

I can't get through the day without eating chocolate. It may make me fat. It may make my symptoms worse. But it makes me feel good. I don't think I could get by without it.
Lara, 21

Food alone can't cure a low mood, but many of us turn to food for comfort. We each have our own idea of the foods that can make us feel happier. Many of the foods we use to cheer ourselves up are connected with childhood. As adults, when we feel down we try to rekindle good feelings by eating foods associated with those times.

For some women with PCOS, the need to eat sugary foods can be a result of their insulin metabolism being out of synch, in the same way that it is for people with diabetes. (For ways to deal with this see Chapter 6.) However, other women with PCOS find that they turn to food they consider to be unhealthy as a way of coping with stress or dealing with difficult emotions.

Pete Cohen from Lighten Up points out that there is no such thing as an unhealthy food, only an unhealthy attitude towards food. If you can change your attitude, you can enjoy a healthy diet without feeling deprived or frustrated, and you can deal with your emotions in a more positive way.

Many women comfort-eat with foods they normally 'ban'. But banning just makes things worse. If you ban a food, all you do is think about it. If someone says 'don't think of a pink elephant' what comes into your head? It's the same with banned foods. You need to understand that food is not the enemy. You shouldn't think of certain foods as unhealthy, or feel guilty when you eat a food you think should be banned – you just need to learn how to choose wisely about the foods you eat.

EATING TO BEAT STRESS

Do you reach for a soothing milky drink when you need to calm down, hope that an extra strong coffee will lift you from your lethargy, or rely on munching chocolate to keep your energy up? Do you find that you start well with a light, healthy breakfast but as stresses build up during the day you lose your resolve and overeat till bedtime?

Every time I have a deadline at work, the digestive biscuits come out – along with several milky coffees. Sometimes I'll eat a whole packet of biscuits in one afternoon. I spend the rest of the day feeling guilty and overeating because I feel I've let myself down, and feel I may as well carry on.
Connie, 30

I usually eat a healthy breakfast, but by 4 p.m. I'm starving. I'll reach for anything to keep me going, and I usually keep reaching for something until I go to bed. I know it's wrong and I'm eating too much, but I get weak and can't think clearly if I don't get my food fixes to help me through the day.
Stacey, 44

Life is stressful. Life with PCOS can be very stressful. So how do many of us cope when we allow stress to overwhelm us? We look for an antidote to our emotional pain. It can be friends, work, fun, alcohol, sex or drugs, but for many women it is food. And too much food leads to poor health and weight gain, which in turn leads to – you've guessed it – lots more stress and unhappiness. But why does stress make you want to eat?

Your stress hormones – cortisol and corticotrophin-releasing hormone – peak first thing in the morning, at around 6 to 8 a.m. It is during this time that you feel most alert and able to concentrate. By mid-morning they are starting to decline (coffee-craving time) and by mid-afternoon you can actually feel a drop in energy and concentration – usually around 3 to 4 p.m. Your body is preparing to rest and sleep after a day of activity. Your stress hormones reach their lowest levels when you sleep, and start gearing up again around 2 a.m.

It's natural to feel less energy as the day progresses. Unfortunately, though, we don't live in tune with our natural stress rhythms. At the time of the day when we should be starting to wind down, many of us start up another day's worth of activity – deadlines, traffic, dinners and countless domestic errands and responsibilities. Stressed and tired, many of us, faced with all these burdens, seek momentary pleasure and relief with food between the hours of 3 p.m. and midnight, although some of us may notice a loss of energy as early as 10 a.m.

Eating Late at Night

According to new research, binge eaters, vegetarians, alcoholics and reformed smokers are all at their most vulnerable at night time. A report published in the journal *Personality* found that people who go to bed late are more likely to suffer from bulimia. In addition, bulimia is more prevalent in the winter months with longer nights. The report explains that lack of light is the most likely explanation: 'Dimly lit settings make people less inhibited and undermine their control.'

If you find that your resolve weakens in the evening or late at night, try to make sure you eat enough during the day so that you aren't ravenous by the evening. Don't skip breakfast, lunch or your mid-morning or mid-afternoon snacks. If you do feel tempted to overeat when night draws in, distract yourself by taking a walk, having a bath, reading a book, chatting to a friend on the phone or anything else that doesn't involve eating. Limit your alcohol intake, and if you dine out choose light, healthy options. You may find it helpful to have an eating curfew, say 8 p.m., when you brush your teeth and decide to stop eating for the day. Chewing gum or sucking a mint can also help to give you the feeling of a psychological 'full-stop' on food.

The trouble with stress-related eating and overeating later in the day is that it is one of the biggest causes of weight gain in women. And it's particularly unhelpful if you have PCOS – we've already seen how both stress and excess weight can trigger symptoms. If you do find yourself turning to food for comfort to help you get through the day, or think that your difficult relationship with food is making it hard for you to manage your weight and follow a healthy eating plan, it is crucial that you understand the link between food and mood so that you can move towards a more healthy attitude to eating.

FOOD AND MOOD

I spend a lot of my time thinking, 'What did I do to deserve PCOS. Why me?' And the worst thing about it all is that it's out of my hands. I can't fix it. I'm stuck with it. I'm not going to be cured. This makes it so hard for me to keep going. The only thing that keeps me hanging on is food. Eating foods I love makes me feel better and helps me manage.
Sara, 29

There is a reason why some foods can make you feel happier, and why others can make you depressed. Within your brain, chemicals help transmit messengers from one nerve cell to another. Two such chemicals

– serotonin and norepinephrine – affect the way you feel. Your body makes these endorphins from the food you eat – so you can, to a certain extent, raise the levels of these chemicals by eating certain foods.

Not surprisingly, the main sources of endorphins are sugary, carbohydrate-rich foods. This is why you may feel happier after those biscuits, cakes, chocolates, sugary cereals, white bread, white rice and pasta.

As you know, the problem with eating such high-sugar foods is that their sugars enter your bloodstream very quickly and cause, along with a rush of serotonin, a rush of insulin, something women with PCOS need to avoid. If there is a sudden rise in sugar levels, the insulin breaks it down quickly, leading to a drop in both sugar and endorphin. This leaves you feeling worse than before.

Many women with PCOS are particularly sensitive to the swings in endorphins:

I can't eat chocolate on its own. Within minutes I feel agitated, moody and aggressive.
Anthea, 25

I really love eating white bread and jam, and a cream tea is my idea of heaven, but before I eat it I have to decide if I am prepared to pay the price. I know that I'll feel terrible for the rest of the day.
Janine, 37

Feeling good isn't just a matter of including serotonin and norepinephrine foods in your eating plan. You need vitamins and minerals – deficiencies may make you feel low. If you feel low you may eat more sugary foods to try to boost your mood, setting up a vicious cycle of nutritional deficiency and depression. (See Chapter 6 for more on this and how you can help yourself.)

The effect of food on our emotions, and how our emotions are affected by the food we eat, is an emerging science. We need to recognize and appreciate that the relationship between food and our emotions is yet another key to healthy eating.

Food is a powerful tool you can use to improve not just your physical health but your emotional health, too. In the words of Judith Wurtzman, PhD (who, along with Richard Wurtzman, MD at the Massachusetts Institute of Technology, was the first to link food with mood when they found that the sugar and starch in carbohydrate foods boost serotonin levels): 'With all that we now know about the food/mind/mood connection you can begin to select food that will ... modify your moods and ... make you a more effective, motivated and perhaps even more contented individual.'[1]

Dieticians Sally Wharmby and Claire Mellors, who run a PCOS clinic at Queens Medical Centre in Nottingham, say 'Women with PCOS should not underestimate the powerful effect food can have, not just on your physical health but on your emotional health too. You are eating not just to improve your symptoms and your chance of health in the future, you are eating to feel happier and more content.'

PCOS and Eating Disorders

Some days I eat really healthily. Then on other days I get so fed up of feeling tired and having acne and irregular periods that I eat all day long. If I can I'll vomit before I go to bed. I know it isn't good for me and I know it will make my symptoms worse, and each time I say 'never again', but it keeps happening.
Lisa, 34

The aim of this book is to make food work for you, but the issue of control over food can be problematic for some women with PCOS. If you feel unhappy with the way you look and feel, there is the risk that you will go about trying to change this in the wrong way. You may try to starve yourself into a dangerously malnourished condition and hide your body behind loose and baggy clothes. Even when very thin, you may think you are overweight and become terrified of gaining any more. In the grip of anorexia, you may be willing to sacrifice everything to stay thin, even your health.

Alternatively, you could find yourself bingeing on massive amounts of food and then vomiting or using laxatives to rid yourself of them. You may go on strict diets and exercise obsessively. Bulimia sufferers' weight appears normal but is maintained with bizarre eating patterns. Frequent vomiting distends your stomach. Your teeth become like that of a much older woman because of the stomach acids that have worn away the enamel. Stomach and mouth ulcers are also likely. As for someone who is anorexic, your hair, nails, teeth and bones will suffer without the correct nutrients.

Overeating, or bingeing without purging, is another form of eating disorder. What is dangerous is not the occasional indulgence but indulgence on a regular basis which will eventually lead to excess weight. Overeating puts a strain on your kidneys, liver, intestines, digestive system and heart. Everything you do becomes tiring and you put your health at risk both now and in the future.

If you have an eating disorder, your body does not get the nutrients it needs to maintain a healthy menstrual cycle. Stresses which have been found to contribute to eating disorders and disruption of the menstrual cycle include low self-esteem about being female or becoming a mother yourself.[2] For instance, if you have grown up being told that women are inferior, on some level you may want no part of being female. In some cases these negative feelings may contribute towards unhealthy eating patterns. There may be suppressed rage at your parents, or guilt and fear about your need for parental care and protection and fear of losing this protection. As you grow up, such negative feelings can manifest in low self-esteem and eating disorders, which – because they stop you ovulating and make you more 'androgenous' – could be viewed as an attempt to 'halt' becoming a mature woman. There may also be deeper emotional hurts from your past or your present, like a partner leaving you, a job loss or your parents dying, which create stress that can manifest in poor eating habits and a disrupted menstrual cycle.

When my hair started thinning and my periods stopped I worried that it might be to do with my busy lifestyle. I'm not very good at taking it easy or expressing emotions. I'm a strong believer in the mind/body connection with PCOS. I don't think my PCOS is self-inflicted, but I had a lot of emotional hurt inside me from the death of both my parents in a car crash when I was just 15. Finally, after one weekend of self-reflection and a lot of crying I started to have stomach cramps and a heavy bleed. It was as if I was letting go of all the pain and hurt I had been repressing. Doctors were amazed at how, overnight, my periods returned. I have learned a lot about myself and how internalizing emotions can make my symptoms worse.
Trisha, 38

Most dieticians, nutritionists and psychologists agree that our attitudes towards food are influenced by our upbringing, most especially by the mother figure, and that issues of control over others, control over ourselves and other psychological factors such as not wanting to face adulthood are the main triggers of eating disorders, which are intensified by media hype.

Experts differ as to whether there is a link between eating disorders and PCOS. Several studies suggest that as many as 60 per cent of women with bulimia also have PCO/S,[3] but other research suggests that there is no link between the two.[4] Since many women with PCOS have problems controlling their weight, an association would not be surprising. Bear in mind, too, that bingeing and starving can trigger insulin resistance.

Eating Disorder or Disordered Eating?

Many women with PCOS feel that the condition has made them more vulnerable to eating disorders or disordered eating patterns.

You may have tried to control your weight to ease your symptoms, and perhaps this has led to an eating disorder.

I was diagnosed with PCOS in my early thirties and told to lose weight to improve my symptoms. I wanted to lose weight and tried every diet in the book. Nothing worked, so I simply stopped eating. I got so ill that I had to go into hospital.
Kate, 40

When I was an overweight 15 year old my doctor told me that the only way I could get my symptoms under control (absent periods, hair on my face and chest, and acne) was to lose weight. My symptoms improved so dramatically when I lost weight that I just took things too far. Now I associate weight gain with being fat, hairy and unattractive. I'm still scared to eat normally and will do anything – vomiting, taking laxatives, not eating at all – to keep my weight down.
Jean, 29

You may not be anorexic or bulimic but still have an unhealthy attitude towards food. Full-blown eating disorders like anorexia and bulimia tend to receive the most attention because of their shock value. For years now we have become used to hearing about anorexia and bulimia. Lost in the shuffle, however, are women with less severe cases of dysfunctional eating. They don't take it so far, but they hate their bodies just as much.

Dysfunctional eating is defined in terms of how much time you spend thinking about food and weight. Women with eating disorders think about food almost all the time. Dysfunctional eaters think about food more than is considered normal. A poor body image is often combined with dysfunctional eating to keep weight low, and obsessive exercise to burn calories. There is an irrational fear of gaining weight, and one's happiness and sense of self-worth are based on food and exercise choices.

Are you constantly on a diet, always switching from one new fad to the next one? If food isn't about enjoying a nice meal or eating to refuel your body, but has started to take up more time and attention than it should, you could have an unhealthy relationship with food. A woman's relationship with food is often very complicated, whether PCOS is involved or not. But knowing that weight gain can make your PCOS symptoms worse, along with the fact that insulin resistance and a slower metabolism means you put on weight more easily, could make you vulnerable to dysfunctional eating patterns.

It can be hard not to see your body as the enemy when you have PCOS. Just as dieters constantly think about forbidden foods, you may find yourself thinking constantly about foods you know won't help you. Denying yourself food, then binge-eating, comfort-eating or simply thinking about planning your food can give you a feeling of control over your body, your life and emotional situations you are in, even if that control makes you feel unwell and unhappy in the long term. The relief this feeling of control over your life gives you can be so powerful that it becomes addictive, and starts a cycle of emotional eating that can be hard to break.

In the long run this cycle – apart from the damaging effects of making you feel miserable and a slave to your food – will cause problems with your PCOS. If you have disordered eating routines you won't be getting all the nutrients you need to balance your hormones and your blood sugar, and this will make your symptoms worse. You will also be increasing the risk of long-term health problems such as diabetes, heart disease and infertility. And weight-management will be harder because unhealthy eating patterns confuse your metabolic rate so that when you do eat normally you store a greater proportion of what you eat as fat.

If you have been diagnosed with PCOS and start to fast, binge, diet or yo-yo diet, not only can this create nutritional deficiencies but it can also disrupt the delicate insulin mechanism further and actually trigger symptoms of PCOS. So an unhealthy attitude towards food not only stops you feeling better, but can actually trigger PCOS in those with a genetic predisposition. If you have PCO or PCOS you need to tackle disordered eating patterns before you tackle the PCO/S.

SEEKING HELP

If you comfort-eat, or eating makes you feel guilty, or you feel uncomfortable eating in public, or are going from one fad diet to another, or just don't think about food in the normal way, these are all warning signs that you could be developing an unhealthy relationship with food. It is important that you get help and support to reduce the health risks associated with a poor diet.

I'm on the Pill – I have abnormal periods if I'm not. I get the hair on the face and the belly and severe water retention. I also have bulimia.

Not until I bought a computer last year, got on the internet and happened across a medical website that dealt with PCOS did I discover that I am not alone and I have a real reason for being fat! I have found a new doctor who is giving me advice about diet and exercise in combination with medication, and things are looking up. I'm also talking to friends and family more about my eating problems, and everyone is on my side. I'm taking saw palmetto, and my acne and facial hair have definitely improved. Finding out that there were others like me, enlisting the support of family and friends and making grown-up choices about food have made a huge difference. I am still not completely sane yet, but I'm feeling hopeful for the first time in my life.

I am unsure if this is all because I finally know what is wrong with me – it isn't all my fault, I have PCOS and this may partly explain my bulimia – or because I have started to pay attention to the food I eat, but I feel so much better. With everything we PCOSers have to watch out for – heart problems, diabetes, infertility – it is nice to think I may get this under control!
Chloe, 40

Before making any dietary changes, you need to get your relationship with food back on track. Starting to have treatment for PCOS if you are not already doing so can be helpful. You can share your eating problems with other women who have gone through the same thing by joining a support group in your area or on the internet. You can also get support from eating disorders organizations and specialist centres (see Chapter 12). Your doctor can put you in touch with a dietician if you think this will be helpful, or help you find a counsellor who specializes in eating problems. If your unhealthy attitude towards food comes from a particular PCOS-related symptom such as acne, hirsutism or infertility causing low self-esteem, body image problems or depression, you may want to ask for a counsellor who can help you with these issues. If you don't want to ask your doctor for this kind of help, you can do some research to find a suitable counsellor yourself. If you don't think your eating problems are PCOS-related but caused by other life issues, you may want a counsellor who is a specialist in, say, family relationships, marriages, coping with violence and so on.

You may also find the five-step plan below helpful. You'll see that the focus here isn't on diet but on understanding your relationship with food so that you can move towards more healthy attitudes. It's also about self-esteem and body image. Part of regaining a healthy attitude towards food is separating food from negative feelings about yourself. Once you begin to do that, you can feel free to eat what is good for you without feeling deprived.

Warning: If your eating patterns are so out of control that the quality of your life is being affected, it is important that you seek medical advice immediately.

RESTORING THE BALANCE

1) Step One: Relaxation

If thinking about food makes you feel anxious, one of the most thoroughly tested anti-anxiety techniques is relaxation. Not only can relaxation calm the physical signs of anxiety such as a rapid heart beat and sweating, it can also calm you mentally and emotionally. Sally Wharmby and Claire Mellors recommend that women with PCOS and emotional eating problems find ways to ease tension and relax, such as 'phoning a friend, having a bath or listening to your favourite music'.

Anxiety is nature's alarm system to help you cope with stressful situations, but too much anxiety can affect your symptoms and your long-term health. High levels of the stress hormone cortisol, released by the adrenal gland, are associated with many of the symptoms of PCOS. According to one US study, while chronic anger increases the risk of heart disease in men, for women it's anxiety that poses this risk.

There are many ways to relax; you need to find what works best for you. Sitting down in a quiet place where you won't be disturbed, taking slow deep breaths and gently clenching and relaxing all your muscles, starting with your toes and moving up to your shoulders, face and jaw can be an enjoyable and easy way to relax. Or you could try the 'any time, any place' technique of mentally scanning your body for tension points, exaggerating the tension and then letting it go. You may prefer to go for a long walk or listen to calming music. If it relaxes you, frees you from tension and clears your mind so that you can start to think about what you want to achieve, then do it.

When you feel a food craving, slowing down your breathing can help. The minute you become anxious your breathing becomes more shallow and rapid, increasing your anxiety. To interrupt this, take slow deep breaths through your nostrils and focus on your diaphragm as it moves up and down. As a rough guide, aim for four or five seconds to breathe in and the same for breathing out.

Pete Cohen from Lighten Up suggests putting your knife and fork down in between mouthfuls and taking a deep breath, so you don't bolt down your food in an anxious way that contributes to indigestion and overeating.

Meditation can also ease anxiety and stress – perhaps because it shuts off your mind and allows your body to relax. You don't need to join a class or do any fancy techniques: just sit upright, close your eyes and focus on your breathing. It might help to say a word such as 'calm', 'contentment' or 'peace' quietly to yourself. If unwanted thoughts about food intrude, simply acknowledge them and then let them go, as if your thoughts are like grains of sand running through your fingers. For the best results aim to meditate for 10 to 20 minutes twice a day. (See Chapter 12 for further information.)

Other ways of managing anxiety include talking to a friend, partner or family member, to help you put things in perspective. You could also imagine the worse-case scenario – you'll see that many of your worst fears are not real possibilities but exaggerations that don't stand up to this kind of 'reality check'.

Food was a bit like a sedative I'd use whenever I felt anxious or worried about my PCOS or other problems in my life. Now I use breathing exercises to calm me. They also help me see that the great majority of the time it's my reaction to a situation, and not the situation itself, that is causing the stress.
Josie, 36

2) Step Two: Awareness

I eat several packets of crisps and lots of sweet snacks like muffins and cookies every day. It started out as something to reward myself at the end of the day. Now I don't want to eat so much anymore because I'm gaining weight fast, which isn't good for my symptoms, but I find I can't stop.
Becky, 19

Overeating in response to stress and anxiety can often become a habit, but like any habit it can be broken. Becoming aware of when you eat, what you eat and how you eat can help you replace negative habits with positive ones, so that if you choose to enjoy the odd chocolate bar, glass of wine, etc., it will be a positive choice that you really appreciate rather than caused by underlying emotional tensions which make the treat ultimately unsatisfying.

Your Food and Mood Diary

It may seem like a chore keeping a food and mood diary but, hopefully, you will begin to enjoy putting some thought into what you are eating and how you are feeling. Remember this diary isn't about controlling your diet, it's about understanding your eating habits.

A diary works best if kept in a clear and methodical manner. Find yourself a conveniently sized notebook you can carry around with you. It works best to write down what you eat and drink at the time you have it. Sometimes at the end of the day it can be hard to remember.

Your diary notes could include the following –

How hungry you are before eating
How you feel physically
How you feel mentally/emotionally
What you eat
What you drink
How hungry you are after eating
How you feel physically
How you feel mentally/emotionally

– as well as examples of physical symptoms such as fatigue, headache, stomach ache, backache or weakness. Examples of emotional or mental symptoms may include: anxiety, irritability, forgetfulness, lack of concentration, restlessness, anger, sadness, boredom, tearfulness or happiness.

Rating symptoms provides you with a way of comparing them and assessing your feelings from one day to the next. You may want to give each symptom a score on a scale of 1 to 5, where 5 is the worst possible feeling and 1 is very mild.

Discovering what food means to you and uncovering your relationship with it will help you understand yourself better. Look honestly at how you use food and how much of it you really eat. If you really want to come to terms with your eating, for two weeks or more write down everything you eat, where you eat it and how you were feeling at the time. This exercise breaks through denial and helps you come to terms with what you are actually eating. You can't address your eating habits until you have looked squarely at the issues around food. You may be able to do this alone, or you may need the help of your doctor, dietician or counsellor.

Becoming more aware of your feelings when you eat will also help you become more attuned to hunger signals. Many women with PCOS and disordered eating have lost the ability to judge when they are actually hungry, and don't know what their bodies need.

Sometimes I just hate the sight of myself in the mirror. I feel fat and unfeminine, and it's even worse when my acne flares up too. I eat when I'm angry. I eat when I'm stressed. I eat when I'm sad. I eat when I'm lonely. I'm never hungry but I always want to eat.
Sophia, 29

Not being able to recognize true hunger signals often stems from not focusing fully on eating. We all do this sometimes. How often do you find yourself popping something into your mouth without thinking about it? The problem with this is if you are not concentrating on your food you don't notice when you are full or have had enough, and by the time you do it is usually too late and you feel guilty because you have overindulged, and feel bloated and overfull.

The next time you want to eat, ask yourself if you are really hungry. If you aren't sure whether you are hungry, you probably aren't. Ask yourself if anything other than food, like a walk, a chat, a hug, would satisfy you instead. If you *are* hungry, a useful tip from the Lighten Up team is to smell your food first. 'Smell is the sense most directly linked to the brain, and it's your sense of smell that will help you get back in touch with what your body really needs,' says Pete Cohen. You might also try drinking a glass of water, as thirst sometimes gets confused with hunger.

When you do eat, take your time between mouthfuls and really think about what you are eating. Slow down. Make eating an event and savour every mouthful. You'll notice that you recognize when you are full sooner, and you'll also notice when you are eating foods that you don't really enjoy. You may even notice that many of the foods you thought you couldn't live without – fast foods and snacks – don't actually taste that good. If you think you want to eat more after a meal, wait 15 minutes and then ask yourself again. It usually takes that amount of time for the brain to register fullness. You'll probably find that your stomach is full, it is your mouth that wants more.

3) Step Three: Focus

Becoming more aware of why you eat, what you eat and whether you are enjoying what you eat will help you build a healthier relationship with food. It will also help you get to the next stage: appreciating that food has far more uses than simply the negative 'making you fat'. Food gives you good skin, hair and teeth as well as a healthy metabolism and the energy to function well and enjoy life.

If you eat the wrong kinds of food you won't feel so good and you will put on weight, whether you have PCOS or not. This isn't about dieting or eating to lose weight. This is about going back to basics, learning about a healthy diet and approaching food in a new way.
Sally Wharmby and Claire Mellors, dieticians, Queens Medical Centre, Nottingham

Focus your thoughts on how your PCOS symptoms will improve through healthier eating habits. This book will have helped you realize how important good food is for women with PCOS, and you know by now that some foods are better than others. The next time you are tempted to eat something which you know is going to lead to poor health, weight gain and a worsening of your symptoms, ask yourself if you will really enjoy it. Wouldn't it be better to choose the healthier alternative?

I was 18 when I was diagnosed with PCOS. I was slowly putting on the pounds and couldn't figure it out. I was totally shocked. I continued to gain the pounds and became very depressed. I finally decided to do something about it. It wasn't going to be easy. My height is 5'5, so 15 stone (210 lb)

really shows – but I was determined. I started an exercise programme, running 6 miles a week, and went on a low-fat diet. It has now been five months and I weigh 11 st 6 (160 lb). I was a size 18–20; now I am a 14. I feel so much better about myself and I still want to lose another 30 lb. Believe me, it is the hardest thing to walk away from food. But I simply remind myself that losing weight will make me feel and look better.
Gillian, 24

A few years ago my eating was all over the place. I lived on junk food and sugary snacks. My periods were non-existent, my hair was lifeless and dull, my skin dry and I had no energy – even getting up the stairs was an effort. I can honestly say that changing my eating habits for the better has changed my life. When I wake up in the morning I can't wait to start the day. I feel healthy and energetic.
Angie, 38

4) Step Four: Regaining Control

Whatever relationship you have with food, one thing most disordered eaters have in common is that they use food as a form of control. This control can appear as constant dieting, guilty overeating, pretending to have a food allergy or to be a vegetarian so that you can avoid eating, or even blaming PCOS for your overeating.

The way people relate to food seems to represent how they exercise control in their lives. If everything else in their lives is in chaos, the best form of control open to them is to control what they eat.
Dr Janis Smith, consultant clinical psychologist

Symptoms of PCOS can be frightening and overwhelming, and many women use food for feelings of comfort and control. We encourage our clients to look for other ways to find comfort apart from the quick fix food offers. This can lead to new hobbies, interests and friendships. When you find time for yourself to do the things you enjoy, your self-esteem improves ... many of our clients say that they feel great and haven't time to think so much about food now that they have other interests.
Sally Wharmby and Claire Mellors

Once you become aware of the fact that you are using food to enhance feelings of comfort and control, you are better placed to make positive changes and break out of old habits. You can start looking for opportunities to make changes and for other ways to comfort yourself. For instance, you could start eating pleasurable foods only when you have time to really enjoy them; you could stop eating when you have had enough; you could snack on fruit instead of chocolate. You could phone a friend instead of eating a packet of crisps, go for a walk instead of reaching for the biscuits, watch a favourite video or give someone a hug instead of stocking up on cakes.

Making these kinds of changes may involve working on your self-esteem. We operate on the belief that if you really want something you should have it – but you need to take control and enjoy eating it in moderation. To be able to do that you need to feel good about yourself.
Olivia Verity, Lighten Up

You may think that you are treating yourself when you eat comfort foods, but if it leads to weight gain and a worsening of your symptoms, is this really a treat? If you find yourself comfort-eating on a regular basis, your self-esteem could be low. The feeling may be triggered by PCOS or by a PCOS symptom such as like weight gain, hirsutism or acne making you feel that you aren't good enough or attractive enough in the eyes of the world. Or it can be triggered by any experience which makes you dislike the person you are. Whatever your trigger, low self-esteem has a negative impact on your eating habits.

Whether a woman has PCOS or not, low self-esteem often manifests itself in unhealthy eating patterns. If PCOS is the case, a woman is very vulnerable to low esteem, especially if appearance, weight or fertility are negatively affected.
Dr Adam Carey, Centre for Nutritional Medicine, London

If you often feel bad about yourself because you have PCOS, or for some other reason, this can be a hard habit to break out of. It can also stop you taking care of yourself. The first thing you need to understand is that you are an OK person. You deserve the best, and that includes eating things that are good for you. The self-esteem boosting suggestions below may be helpful.

Use affirmations	Positive statements you repeat to yourself over and over again until they sink in are a powerful way to boost self-esteem. Whenever you hear yourself saying, 'I can't,' 'I won't,' 'I shouldn't,' 'I ought to' or 'What if?', replace them with positive ones in the present tense: 'I can lose weight.' 'I feel confident.' 'There is nothing to fear. I can handle it.'
Confront your fear	The only way to get rid of fear is to go out and face it. The fear of doing something is often worse than the discomfort of doing it. If you are worried that you won't be able to lose weight or eat healthily, the best thing to do is to try. If you are worried that PCOS will destroy your health, take action to prevent that happening.
Stop trying to be perfect	Remind yourself that you have a right to be assertive, to have opinions and emotions and be successful. Just because you have PCOS doesn't mean that you are any less of a person. You also have the right to make mistakes and change your mind. There will be times when you won't eat healthily. It's not a big deal. Just start eating healthily again tomorrow.
Avoid put-downs	Self-critical language doesn't help anyone. Use self-respectful language, avoid exaggeration and focus on your behaviour, NOT you as a person. For example, not 'I'm too fat for this dress,' but 'This dress isn't right for me, let me try another size.'

Respect your body	Whatever your size, learn to respect the body you have, one day at a time. Women who respect their bodies and like themselves are irresistible and fun to be around, regardless of their dress size.
Play to your strengths and don't focus on your weaknesses	Don't spend hours shopping for clothes you hope will hide your body. Shop for clothes that will highlight your hair colour or your eyes.
Give yourself lots of non-food treats	Spend more time pampering yourself, especially during stressful times. Have a soothing bath or a facial, get your hair cut, visit old friends, go to the theatre, set aside time to curl up with a good book or magazine.
Get support	Turn to those people who enjoy your strengths and accept your weaknesses, not those who put you down. If you always come away feeling good after seeing someone, see more of them.
Be yourself	Don't play a role for someone else. Do you really think you need to lose weight, or are you trying to match someone else's idea of perfection? Keep an eye on your goals, too, and make sure they are what *you* want.
Give yourself time	We all need quality time with ourselves. Learn to value and enjoy solitude and your own company and thoughts.
Say no	Start to say no more often. Tell yourself firmly but often that it is important to consider your own needs as well as other people's. For example, you come home after a long, hard day at work when your friend calls and asks you to

baby-sit. Instead of feeling obliged and guilty, tell your friend that if she'd given you more notice you would have been happy to help, but tonight you need time to relax and unwind.

Don't hide away — Don't try to hide or cover up the fact that you have PCOS. It is nothing to be ashamed of. Encourage the people in your life who care about you to understand the condition so that you can all work together.

5) Make the Decision to Change

When you have started to become aware of how food affects your mood, that there is a new way to approach food and that you deserve to be eating good food, this brings you to the final stage: Doing it.

I exhibit most of the classical signs of PCOS – looking back I think that my doctor back home should have investigated the possibility of PCOS – when I was 15 I had very bad acne and excruciatingly painful periods. I didn't find out that I had PCOS until I was 28. I know that PCOS isn't entirely to blame for my weight problems. I still get depressed and binge eat, and I should be doing something about it.
Caroline, 30

You may have started to adjust your life to your symptoms, but deep down the thought of change can be overwhelming. Moving from the intention to make changes to actually doing it can be a big challenge, whether you have PCOS or not. 'You can be motivated,' says Judith Verity from Lighten Up, 'but not motivated enough to change. If you really want to look and feel better, if you are really motivated to change it will happen.'

Change is scary and you may well feel a bit nervous and unsettled at first. Many women with weight to lose who are experiencing fertility problems find the necessary motivation to lose weight when their doctor tells them that this will increase their chances of getting pregnant. Whether or not you are trying for a baby, you can always find your motivation by reminding yourself constantly that many things about PCOS are uncertain, but one thing isn't: a healthy diet will improve your symptoms, protect your future health, increase the power of any medication you take and help you enjoy your life.

However severe your PCOS symptoms, a healthy, balanced diet has to be part of any action plan to treat your symptoms, get you out of a low mood and help you lose weight, if you need to. Try to combine careful self-reflection with finding out what food means to you, then go ahead and make gradual step-by-step changes according to the guidelines here and in Chapter 3. If the going gets tough, never forget that by taking charge of your diet and making positive changes you're doing all you can to improve your symptoms and protect your health in the future.

Stress-proofing Your Diet

Stress-proofing your diet can help you at those times when you know you are most vulnerable and when you need to adapt your eating to life's routine stressors (work deadlines, rush hour, family dinners, colds, etc.).

– Plan ahead with a daily eating schedule, and know what you are going to eat for your mid-afternoon and mid-evening snacks. Without planning you make yourself vulnerable to overeating, especially at the most trying time for comfort eaters, 3 p.m. to midnight. This need not become another stress. Make out healthy shopping lists, keep healthy snacks on your desk at work and in the cupboard at home, and find out which local restaurants serve healthy foods if you're going to be dining out so you can suggest them as good venues.
– Don't skip breakfast. This will just make you eat too much later in the day.
– Plan a mid-morning snack for around 3 hours after breakfast – ideally a protein source like yogurt and a piece of fruit.
– Eat your mid-afternoon snack about 3 hours after you eat lunch. This could include protein as well as carbohydrates, and should be low in

fat. Examples include soup with crackers, cottage cheese and fruit, yogurt and fruit.

– Try to eat most of your calories before 5 p.m., and don't eat too much after 8 p.m.

– Sometimes, however much you plan ahead, things change. You have to be able to adapt your eating routine to our fast-paced society. Keep your cupboards, fridge and freezer well stocked with emergency healthy foods like soup, beans, canned veggies and low-fat frozen meals. Chopped fresh fruit and vegetables make great sandwich fillers and are good to nibble on whenever you feel hungry. If you have to eat out, see page 53 for tips on eating at restaurants. If you find your routine totally disrupted, keep as active as you can and help yourself to fruit, yogurt and made-to-order sandwiches rather than high-fat alternatives.

– Have a little of what you fancy. Don't worry if you feel you need to treat yourself every now and again. An occasional sweet, cake, chocolate or piece of white bread won't hurt. Sometimes these things can cheer you up. A glass of wine or two may be just what you fancy. So go ahead and enjoy it. Remember, everything is good in moderation – just don't get into the habit of turning to alcohol or sugary foods as the only way to relax. The same applies for tea, coffee and chocolate.

– Keep cooking simple. Many comforting foods are easy to prepare, but they needn't be unhealthy. Try soup with beans, low-fat cheese on toast or baked apples with raisins. Keep your meals simple, but don't feel guilty if once in a while you have a ready-prepared meal when you know that cooking would make you feel tired and stressed. Make eating a pleasurable activity. Sit down to eat, include a variety of fresh, colourful and tasty ingredients in your meals, and try to make sure you eat in a peaceful environment.

Supplements

If you have been feeling low for a while, a good multivitamin and mineral might be wise right now to get you back on track. 'Because the amount of nutrients within foods varies enormously and the soil on which the food is grown may be lacking in minerals,' says nutritional therapist and founder of the MIND Food and Mood Project, Amanda Geary, 'taking nutritional supplements may be the only way to obtain what is needed to feel well.' But remember that your body absorbs vitamins and minerals much more efficiently alongside a healthy and balanced diet, so don't see supplements as an alternative to eating well. And don't think about taking large doses of vitamins and minerals in the hope of curing depression – they won't, and could cause serious problems. See your doctor instead.

Exercise

Don't forget the healing power of exercise. It can make you feel happier because it makes your body produce endorphins such as serotonin. It can also help you lose weight by building muscle and speeding up your metabolism, manage your stress hormones and distract you from food. In a situation when you feel hopeless and out of control, exercise can give you feelings of pleasure and control.

EAT WELL AND HAVE FUN

Everything you eat and drink will affect how you feel, and the way you feel affects your food choices. Bear in mind, though, that exactly how food affects mood and your symptoms will vary from one woman to another. You need to find what works best for you. Yet even though we are all different, getting your relationship with food back on track by learning how important a healthy, balanced diet is for physical and emotional health, and then moving towards healthier eating patterns, will, as we've stressed throughout, be of enormous value.

(Turn to Chapter 12 for more help on dealing with self-esteem, eating disorders, and weight-management problems.)

As you know, living with PCOS can be tough. But like any challenge in life there are rewards to be gained. Whether or not you take medication, learning how positive dietary changes can help you take charge of your health will help you improve your physical, mental and emotional well-being, now and in the years to come.

Hopefully this book will have helped you see food as an empowering tool. Food isn't the enemy. It can improve your symptoms, give you energy and make you feel better and think more clearly. It can also be a lot of fun. A delicious and healthy eating pattern is one of life's great pleasures. And you deserve to enjoy it.

Bon appétit!

12

Support and Information: Useful Addresses and Websites

CONTACTS

This is a list of places where you can find out more about PCOS in general, your specific symptoms, and any therapies that can help you deal with PCOS both physically and emotionally. Always send a stamped addressed envelope when you write off to an address, as many of these places are charities or run by volunteers.

The internet is also a huge source of information and support – don't forget that its beauty is that it's international, so you can get great information and help from any of the websites listed throughout this chapter, not just from those organizations based in your own country.

In addition to your doctor's advice, a PCOS support group should be your first port of call. Groups like Verity in the UK or PCOS Support in the US can give you the advice, support and information you need to make informed choices about your diet, weight management, treatment options and healthcare.

UK

PCOS

Verity
52–54 Featherstone Street
London EC1Y 8RT
www.verity-pcos.org.uk

Acne

The Acne Support Group
PO Box 230
Hayes
Middlesex UB4 0UT
020 8561 6868

The Sher System
The Sher System acne helpline is based in London on:
020 7499 4022

Alopecia (Hair Loss)

Hairline International – The Alopecia Patients Society
Lyons Court
1668 High Street
Knowle
West Midlands B93 0LY
01564 775281

Complementary Therapies

British Complementary Medicine Association
www.bcma.co.uk

The Natural Medicine Society
Regency House
97–107 Hagley Road
Edgbaston
Birmingham B16

Counselling

British Association for Counselling
1 Regent Place
Rugby
Warwickshire CV21 2PJ

Depression

Depression Alliance
35 Westminster Bridge Road
London SE1 7JB
020 7633 9929

MIND – Mental Health Charity
15–19 Broadway
London E15 4BQ
020 8522 1728 (Greater London)
0345 660 163 (outside London)

Detox

The Breakspear Hospital
Hertfordshire House
Wood Lane
Hemel Hempstead
Herts HP2 4FD
01442 261333
Medically-supervised nutritional detox programs

Environmental Air Systems
Martin Wells
Sandyhill Cottage
Sandy Lane
Rushmore
Tilford
Farnham
Surrey GU10 2ET

FACT – Food Additives Campaign Team
25 Horsell Road
London N5 1XL

Healthy House
Cold Harbour
Ruscombe, Stroud
Glos GL6 6DA

The Pesticide Trust
Pesticide Exposure Group of Sufferers
Eurolink Centre
49 Effra Road
London SW2 1BZ
020 7274 8895

Society for Environmental Therapy
Mrs H Davidson
521 Foxhall Road
Ipswich IP3 8LW
01473 723552

Smoking Quitline [UK]
0800 002200

Diabetes

British Diabetic Association
10 Queen Anne Street
London W1M 0BD
020 7323 1531

Eating Disorders

Anorexia and Bulimia Care
Tottenham Women's Health Centre
15 Fenhurst Gate
Aughton
Ormskirk
Lancs L39 5ED
01695 422 479

Centre for Eating Disorders
020 7291 4565

Eating Disorders Association
Sackville Place
44 Magdalen Street
Norwich
Norfolk NR3 1JE
0160 362 1414

Overeaters Anonymous
01273 624 712
Nationwide local groups throughout the UK

Endometriosis

The SHE Trust
Simply Holistic Endometriosis
Red Hall Lodge
Red Hall Drive
Bracebridge Heath
Lincoln N4 2JT

Excess Hair

British Association of Electrolysis
01908 695297

Aculight
0800 169 3846
Ring for an information pack

Institute of Electrolysis
01908 695297

Fertility

Foresight
The Association for the Promotion of Pre-Conceptual Care
28 The Paddock
Godalming
Surrey GU7 1XD
01483 427 839

Issue – Infertility Support
509 Aldridge Road
Great Barr
Birmingham B44
0121 344 4414
Fax: 0121 344 4336

Maternity Alliance
45 Beech Street
London EC2P 2LX
020 7588 8582

Miscarriage Association
c/o Clayton Hospital
Northgate
Wakefield
W Yorks WF1 3JS
01924 200 799

National Childbirth Trust
Alexandra House
Oldham Terrace
Acton
London W3 7NH

Natural Family Planning Centre
Birmingham Maternity Hospital
Queen Elizabeth Medical Centre
Edgbaston
Birmingham B15 2TG
0121 627 2698

Massage

British Federation of Massage Practitioners
78 Meadow Street
Preston
Lancs PR1 1TS
01772 881063

Medical Herbalism

The College of Practitioners of Phytotherapy
Bucksteep Manor
Bodle Street Green
Near Hailsham
Sussex BN27 4RJ
01323 834 800

General Council and Register of Consultant Herbalists
32 King Edwards Road
Swansea SA1 4LL
01792 655886

National Institute of Medical Herbalists
56 Longbrook Street
Exeter
Devon EX4 6AH
01392 426022

Ann Walker, PhD MNIMH MCPP
Senior Lecturer in Human Nutrition
School of Food Biosciences
The University of Reading
PO Box 226
Whiteknights
Reading RG6 6AP

Meditation

Transcendental Meditation
Beacon House
Willow Walk
Woodley Park
Skelmersdale
Lancs WN8 6UR
08705 143733
For information about courses in your area

Transcendental Meditation Association
Freepost
London SW1P 4YY
0990 143733
For TM on the NHS your doctor would need to call Norma Sullivan at the TM Communications Office on 08705 143733 to request a doctor's information pack and free video. This will include advice on funding for your GP

Naturopathy

British College of Naturopathy and Osteopathy
General Council and Register of Naturopaths
Frazer House
6 Netherhall Gardens
London NW3 5RR
0207 435 6464

General Council and Register of Naturopaths
Goswell House
2 Goswell Road
Somerset BA16 0JG
01458 840072

Nutrition

British Association of Allergy, Environmental and Nutritional Medicine
PO Box 28
Totton
Southampton
Hants SO40 2ZA

British Association of Nutritional Therapists
27 Old Gloucester Street
London W1N 3XX
0870 6061284

The Centre for Nutritional Medicine
114 Harley Street
London W1N 1AG
020 7224 5053

Institute of Optimum Nutrition
Blades Court
Deodar Road
London SW15 2NU
020 8877 9993

Vegetarian Society
Parkdale
Dunham Road
Altrincham
Cheshire WA14 4QG
0161 928 0793

Vegan Society
Donald Watson House
7 Battle Road
St Leonards-on-Sea
East Sussex TN3 7AA
01424 427 393

Women's Nutritional Advisory Service
01273 487366

Nutritional Therapists

Marilyn Glenville
Nevill Estate
Danegate
Eridge Green
Tunbridge Wells
Kent TN3 9JA
01892 750511
Information line: 0906 7010030
www.marilynglenville.com

Sally Wharmby and Claire Mellors
Senior Dietitians
Dept of Nutrition and Dietetics
C Floor West Block
Queens Medical Centre
Nottingham NG7 2UH
0115 924 9924 x41040

Organic Living

Food for the Future Foundation
51 Trevelyan
Bracknell
Berkshire RG12 8YD
01344 360033

Friends of the Earth
26–28 Underwood Street
London N1 7JQ
0808 800 1111

Greenpeace
30–31 Islington Green
London N1 8XE

Organic Information
PO Box 1503
Poole
Dorset BH14 8YE
01202 715130

Organic Mail-order Services

A&G Organics
01704 831 393

Farm-a-Round
020 7627 4698

Organic Direct
020 7622 3003

Sellers Organic Produce
01751 472249

Simply Organic
0845 1000 444
Nationwide 48-hour delivery service

Healthy Living Products

Air Improvement Centre
020 7834 2834
Air purifiers, ionizers and humidifiers

Andrews Water Treatment
01704 541 578
For water distillers

Aquapure Distillation
020 8892 9010

Freshwater Filter Company
020 8558 7495

Higher Nature
01435 882880

Wholistic Research Company
01954 781074
Can find juicers, water filters and air purifiers for you and deliver them to your door

You can also buy many of these products in the UK at Boots and other chemists, healthfood stores and places such as Comet, Argos, Currys and Dixons, as well as superstores such as Sainsburys Savacentres.

Chemical-free Cleaning Products

The Green People Company Ltd
01444 401444
www.greenpeople.co.uk

The Green Shop
01452 770629

Healthy House
01453 752216

Herbs Hands Healing
01379 608082

Natural Collection
01225 442288

Natural Woman
0117 946 6649

Supplements

Biocare Nutritional Supplements
54 Northfield Road
Kings Norton
Birmingham B30 1JH
0121 433 3727

Bioforce
www.bioforce.com

Health Plus Ltd
Dolphin House
30 Lushington Road
Eastbourne
East Sussex BN21 4LL
01323 737374

The Herbalist's Centre
38 New Cavendish Street
London W1M 7LH
020 7935 0405

Higher Nature Ltd
The Nutritional Center
Burwash Common
East Sussex TN19 7LX
01435 882880

Kombucha Tea Network
The Hollies
Wellow
Bath
BA2 8QJ
01225 833150
www.kombucha.org.uk

The Nutri Centre
Nutrition Supplements
7 Park Crescent
London W1N 3HE
020 7436 5122

Specialist Herbal Supplies
3 Burton Villas
Hove
Sussex BN3 6BR
01273 202401

Viridian Supplements
31 Alvis Way
Daventry
Northants
NN11 5PG
01327 878050

Other companies whose products are well worth trying are Solgar
Vitamins (01442 890355), Lamberts Healthcare (01892 552120) and Quest.
Ask in your local healthfood shop.

Traditional Chinese Medicine (TCM)

Register of Chinese Herbal Medicine
PO Box 400
Middlesex HA9 9NZ
020 7224 0883

Chi Health Centre
1 Lower Grosvenor Place
Victoria
London SW1W 0EJ
020 7233 5566

Harley Street TCM Fertility Clinic & TCM HealthCare
Head Office
101 Bulwer Road
Leytonstone
London E11 1BU
020 8556 8843 or 0208 558 3708
herb@tcm.uk.com

Weight Loss

Lighten Up
46 Staines Road
Twickenham TW2 5AH
0845 603 3456

Vitaline Weight Control Ltd
144 Ashton Road
Manchester M34 3HR
0161 292 4918
Fax: 0161 292 4919
enquiries@vitaline-slimming.com
Popular with women from PCOS support groups

Sally Wharmby and Claire Mellors
Senior Dietitians
Dept of Nutrition and Dietetics
C Floor West Block, Queens Medical Centre
Nottingham NG7 2UH
0115 924 9924 x41040

Well Woman

Healthline
0800 55 57 77
– freephone number provided by the UK Dept of Health. Call this number to find out what treatment is available, and where, on the NHS.

Women's Environmental Network
87 Worship Street
London EC2A 2BE
020 7247 3327
For information on toxins

Women's Health
52 Featherstone Street
London EC1Y 8RT
020 7251 6580

US AND CANADA

PCOS

Polycystic Ovarian Syndrome Association Inc
PO Box 80517
Portland, OR 97280

Acne

American Academy of Dermatology
PO Box 4014
Schaumburg, IL 60168–4014
(847) 330-0230 or (888) 462-3376

Alopecia

Alopecia Support Group
Frank Smith
4488 Poplar Avenue
Dunnam 329
Memphis, TN 381177
(901) 682-1103/(901) 761-0576

American Hairloss Council (AHLC)
401 North Michigan Avenue
Chicago, IL 60611

Body Image

Beyond Dieting
Rhonda Zabrodski
c/o Calgary Counseling Center
Suite 200
940 6th Ave
SW Calgary
Alberta T2P 3T1
(403) 265-4980
208.229.231.93/shape/wgames/gen/shape.bodyimage.html
www.BeyondDieting.com
Deals with body image, self-esteem, food relationships and diet education

Complementary Therapies

National Clearing House for Complementary and Alternative Medicine
PO Box 8218
Silver Spring, MD 20907–8218
1-888-664-6226

Canadian Holistic Medical Association
491 Eglington Avenue West
Apt 407
Toronto
Ontario M5N 1A8
1-416-485-3071

Counselling

Concerned Counselling
Telephone counselling service toll-free within the US on 1-888-415-8255

Depression

Depressives Anonymous
329 E 62nd Street
New York, NY 10021
Send a SAE for free information

National Institute of Mental Health
NIMH Public Inquiries
6001 Executive Boulevard
Rm 8184
MSC 9663
Bethesda MD 20892–9663
(301) 443-4513
Fax (301) 443-4279

National Foundation for Depressive Illness
PO Box 2257
New York, NY 10016
(212) 268-4260

Detox

Center for Environmental Medicine
Dr Allan Lieberman
7510 Northforest Drive
North Charleston, SC 29420
(803) 572 1600

Citizens for a Better Environment
Suite 505
942 Market Street
San Francisco, CA 94102

Environmental Action
1525 New Hampshire Avenue, NW
Washington, DC 20036

Environmental Protection Agency Safe Drinking Water Hotline
(800) 426-4791

Environmental Protection Products, Inc
100 Canary Street
Glen Cove, NY 11542
(800) 444-3563

Friends of the Earth
530 7th Street, SE
Washington, DC 20003
(202) 543-4312

Greenpeace USA
1611 Connecticut Ave, NW
Washington, DC 20009

National Coalition Against the Misuse of Pesticides
530 7th Street
Washington, DC 20003
(202) 543-5450

National Mail-order Water-testing Laboratories
6555 Wilson Mills Road
Cleveland, OH 44143
(800) 458-3330

Diabetes

American Diabetes Association
1701 North Beauregard Street
Alexandria, VA 22311

National Diabetes Information Clearing House (NDIC)
1 Information Way
Bethesda, MD 20892–3560
(301) 654-3810

The Diabetes Research and Wellness Foundation
1206 Potomac Street, NW
Washington, DC 20007
Helpline (888) 321-2219
Office (202) 298-9211
Gives out information sheets, free medical ID bracelets and self-management diaries

Eating Disorders

American Anorexia/Bulimia Association
418 E 76th Street
New York, NY 10021
(212) 734-1114

Eating Disorder Recovery
1-888-520-1700
email: jrust@edrecovery.com

Massachusetts Eating Disorders Association (MEDA)
92 Pearl Street
Newton, MA 02458
(617) 558-1881
email: info@medainc.org

Endometriosis

International Endometriosis Association
8585 N. 76th Place
Milwaukee WI 53223–2600
(800) 992-3636 or (414) 355-2200
Fax (414) 355-6065

Fertility

American Fertility Society (AFS)
2140 11th Avenue South
Suite 200
Birmingham, AL 35205–2800
(205) 933-8494

American Society for Reproductive Medicine
1209 Montgomery Highway
Birmingham, AL 35216–2809
(205) 978-5000

The Fertility Institute
6020 Bullard Avenue
New Orleans, LA 70128
(800) 375-0048

Fertility Research Foundation
1430 Second Avenue
New York, NY 10021
(212) 744-5500

Infertility Network Exchange
PO Box 204
East Meadow, NY 11554
(516) 794-9772

International Council of Infertility Information Dissemination (INCIID)
PO Box 91363
Tucson AZ 91363
(520) 544-9548

Resolve
The National Infertility Association
1310 Broadway Avenue
Somerville, MA 02144
(617) 623 0744

Massage

American Massage Therapy Association
820 Davis Street
Suite 100
Evanston, IL 60210
(312) 761-2682

Medical Herbalism

The American Herb Association
PO Box 673
Nevada City, CA 95959

North American Herbalists Guild
PO Box 1683
Sequel, CA 95073

Naturopathy

Canadian Naturopathic Association
205, 1234 17th Avenue
South West
PO Box 3143
Station C
Calgary, Alberta
1-413-244-4487

Nutrition

American Academy of Nutrition
College of Nutrition
3408 Sausalito
Corona del Mar, CA 92625–1638
(949) 760-6788
Home-study courses in nutrition

American Association of Naturopathic Physicians
PO Box 20386
Seattle
Washington 98102
(206) 323-7610

The American Dietetic Association
216 West Jackson Boulevard
Chicago, IL 60606–6995
(312) 899-0040

American Preventative Medical Association
275 Millway
PO Box 732
Barnstable, ME 02630
(508) 362 4343
Register of doctors sympathetic to the natural approach

American Vegan Society
501 Old Harding Highway
Malaga, NJ 08328

Food and Nutrition Information Center
National Agriculture Library
10301 Baltimore Avenue
Room 304
Beltsville, MD 20705–2351
(301) 504 5719

North American Vegetarian Society
PO Box 72
Dolgeville, NY 13329

Price-Pottenger Nutrition Foundation
PO Box 2614
La Mesa, CA 91943–2614
(619) 574-7763

Organic Living

American College of Health Science
6600-D Burleson Road
Austin, TX 78744

Barlean's Organic Oils
4936 Lake Terrell Road
Ferndale, WA 98248
(800) 445-3529

Center for Science in the Public Interest
Americans for Safe Food
1501 16th St, NW
Washington, DC 20036
(202) 332-9110

Essential MicroPure Water
24100 State Route 9 SE, Bldg. A
Woodinville, WA 98072
(425) 488-9400

Wholelife
89 Fifth Avenue
Suite 600
New York
NY 10003

You can learn about organic food and organic farming from the following non-profit organizations:

Organic Trade Association
(413) 774-7511

Organic Farming Research Foundation
(408) 426-6606

The Land Institute
(913) 823-5376

Community Alliance with Family Farmers
(916) 756-8518

Supplements

Blessed Herbs
109 Barre Plains Road
Oakham, MA 01068
(800) 489-4372

Herbal Magic, Inc
PO Box 70
Forest Knolls, CA 94933
(415) 488-9488

Herbal Pharmacy
PO Box 116
Williams, OR 97544
(541) 846-6262

May Way Trading
Chinese Herb Company
1338 Cypress Street
Oakland, CA 94607
(510) 208 3113

Metagenics
Nutritional Supplements
917 Calle Negocio
San Clemente, CA 92673
(714) 366 0818
(800) 692 9400

Nature's Apothecary
6350 Gunpark Dr 500
Boulder, CO 80301
(303) 581 0288 or 800 999 7422

Uni Key Health Systems
PO Box 7168
Bozeman, MT 59771
800-888-4353
You could also call the International Academy of Compounding
Pharmacists in Sugarland, Texas (713 933 8400 or 800 927 4227). They can
assist you in locating a local pharmacy that specializes in natural
prescriptions.

Traditional Chinese Medicine

American Association of Acupuncture and Oriental Medicine
4101 Lake Boone Trail, Ste. 201
Raleigh, NC 27607
(919) 787 5181

Well Woman

National Women's Health Network
514 10th Street NW
Suite 400
Washington, DC 20004
(202) 628 7814

National Women's Health Resource Center (NWHRC)
120 Albany Street, Suite 820
New Brunswick, NJ 08901
(877) 986-9742

OBGYN.net: The Obstetrics and Gynecology Network
5707 Lakemore
Austin, TX 50100
(512) 418 2922
email: info@obgyn.net

Women's Health Network
224 7th Street, NE
Washington, DC 20003
(202) 543-9222

AUSTRALIA

PCOS

POSAA – Polycystic Ovary Syndrome Association of Australia
PO Box E140
Emerton
NSW 2770
612 4733 4342

Medical Herbalism

National Herbalists Association of Australia
Suite 305
BST House
3 Smail Street
Broadway
New South Wales 2007
61 2 211 6437

Nutrition

Australian College of Nutritional and Environmental Medicine
13 Hilton Street
Beaumaris
VIC 3193
03 9589 6088

Australian Natural Therapists (ANTA)
PO Box 308
Melrose Park
South Australia
61-8-371-3222

Australian Naturopathic Practitioners and Chiropractors Association
1st Floor, 609 Camberwell Road
Camberwell
VIC 3124
03 9889 0488

Liver Cleansing and Natural Weight Control Centre
76 Spring Street
Bondi Junction
NSW 2022
02 9387 8111

Naturopathic Physicians Association of Australia Inc
2 Beaumont Road
Canterbury
VIC 3126
03 9836 8103

Women's Health Advisory Service
Dr Sandra Cabot
PO Box 217
Paddington
NSW 2021
02 4655 8855

HELPFUL WEBSITES

PCOS

info@posaa.asn.au
www.pcosupport.org/
www.pcosupport.org/pcoteen/about.html – PCOTeen is a division of
PCOSA for women in their teens who have PCO/S
www.soulcysters.com
www.pcos.net
www.posaa.asn.au
www.midwivesofwa.org/pcos.htm

Acne

www.healthy.net/LIBRARY/BOOKS/Healthyself.acne.htm
www.m2w3.com/acne/
members.tripod.com/~wildsurvival/index.html
www.stopspot.net – for teenagers dealing with acne

Alopecia

follicle.com/types.html
www.jericho.org/-jericho/_ccc_asg.html

Complementary Therapies

www.bloom.com.au
www.desertessence.com.au

www.holistichealthonline
www.internethealthlibrary.com
www.jurlique.com.au
www.thursdayplantation.com.au

Diabetes

www.diabetes.org
www.mendosa.com/org.htm

Eating Disorders

www.anorexia.org/chat/
www.edrecovery.com
members.aol.com/lacillo/eating.html
www.medainc.org/contact.htm

Endometriosis

www.endometriosisassn.org
www.endometriosis.co.uk
www.shetrust.org.uk

Fertility

www.child.org.uk
natfamplan.co.nz/educationservice.html
fertilethoughts.net/malpani
www.preconception.com
www.fertilityinstitute.com
www.4fertility.com/
www.ein.org
alt.infertility.alternatives
www.kumc.edu/gec/support/miscarri.html
www.womens-health.co.uk/miscarr.htm
www.obgyn.net

www.inciid.org
www.resolve.org

Nutrition

www.patrickholford.com
www.thefooddoctor.co.uk
www.naturopathic.org
www.eatright.org
www.nutricentre.com – for information, mail order and access to
nutritionists and a pharmacist

Organic Living

www.organicfood.co.uk – helpful UK website listing mail order companies
and information about where you can buy organic produce locally.
www.simplyorganic.net
www.foe.co.uk/safer_chemicals (friends of the earth)
www.naturalhealthyliving.com

Well Woman

www.healthywoman.org
www.obgyn.net
www.whas.com.au

Appendix
PCOS – Causes, Symptoms, Treatment

Polycystic Ovary Syndrome (PCOS) (also known as Polycystic ovaries, Stein-Leventhal syndrome, and functional ovarian hyperandrogenism) is a health condition linked with hormone imbalance and insulin resistance which can bring about a raft of symptoms from irregular or absent periods to acne, weight gain, fatigue, depression, hair loss, excess body and facial hair and other, less well-known symptoms. Symptoms can be mild or severe, and can vary widely from woman to woman.

It is thought that 10 per cent of women have this condition, even though many of them may not know it because their symptoms may be misdiagnosed – as PMS or stress, for instance.

The basic cause of PCOS is thought to be the inability of the ovaries to produce the correct balance of hormones. Without the correct hormonal stimulation, the ovaries can't develop or release eggs. This leads to the formation of empty egg follicles on the ovary, known as tiny cysts. *Polycystic* means 'many cysts'.

Polycystic ovaries have a string of these empty follicles around their outside. There are usually 10 or more, each usually measuring 2 to 8 millimetres across. When the ovary is viewed using an ultrasound scan, these features can be seen. Having at least 10 cysts with a thickened *stroma* (the name given to the tissue within the ovary, not the follicles, which are made of *thecal* cells) enables a diagnosis of polycystic ovaries.[1]

PCOS is not an ovarian cyst. Polycystic cysts are different to ovarian cysts, which are usually single and can grow bigger and interfere with ovarian function. In PCOS the string of tiny cysts are thought to be egg follicles which have failed to develop completely to release an egg. Although many people wonder if the cysts are the problem, the truth is they are a symptom, not the cause. They are a consequence of the hormonal imbalance in women with PCOS rather than the cause, and should not be removed by surgery. The cysts seen in PCOS are symptoms of deeper underlying hormonal and metabolic problems. If you get these underlying problems sorted out or improved through changes in diet and, if needed, medication, the cysts can reduce in number.

WHAT CAUSES PCOS?

In 1935, when PCOS was first described as a condition by Drs Stein and Leventhal, there was great debate as to what caused it.[2] Stein and Leventhal thought it was probably due to hormonal imbalance. Today the debate continues, and no one is quite sure what causes PCOS.

Elevated levels of Luteinizing Hormone (LH) have been found in some – but not all – women with PCOS. Elevated levels of testosterone are also associated with PCOS and its symptoms. Testosterone inhibits ovulation and causes menstrual irregularity. But the general consensus is that inappropriate levels of LH and testosterone are, again, symptoms rather than cause of PCOS.

Recent research into the cause of PCOS has focused on why some women with PCOS have elevated levels of insulin. It is probable that the elevated insulin levels found in women with PCOS do promote androgen production by the ovaries and contributes to the menstrual disturbances common in women with PCOS, but, as not all women with PCO/S have elevated levels of insulin, it is not the single cause of the problem.

PCOS is a complex disorder generated by a number of factors. It is well known that PCOS seems to run in families, which has led scientists to suggest that the genes controlling androgen and insulin production may play the main role in PCOS.[3] However, other genetic factors may affect the type and severity of the symptoms experienced as well. In addition, environmental issues such as diet, lifestyle, weight and pollution also play important roles in the development and control of symptoms.

WHAT ARE THE SYMPTOMS?

The following symptoms – overweight, irregular or absent periods, acne, infertility and an overgrowth of facial or body hair – are thought to be the 'classic' signs of PCOS which doctors look out for. Yet a number of groups have looked at the symptoms patients present to their doctors and reported that there are a range of symptoms associated with PCOS, including the five mentioned above but also fatigue, joint pain, hair loss (alopecia), tender breasts, bloating, diabetes with insulin resistance, mood swings and depression.[4]

Other PCOS symptoms include:

❈ pelvic pain
❈ breast pain
❈ abdominal pain
❈ dizziness
❈ increased tendency to faint

A woman with PCOS can have any single one or a combination of these symptoms, and symptoms tend to get worse over time and with weight gain.

Let's look at the more common symptoms in more detail:

Irregular or absent periods These are defined as a menstrual cycle of fewer than 21 days or greater than 35 days, or with more than four days' variation from month to month. The menstrual cycle may

be consistently irregular with long gaps –
known as oligomenorrhea – or non-existent
– known as amenorrhea. This often results
in either irregular ovulation or no ovulation
(known as anovulation). It is possible to have
a regular menstrual cycle and not ovulate.
All women at the start and end of their
reproductive lives, and occasionally during,
have menstrual cycles when no ovulation
occurs.

Facial and body hair

This is known as hirsutism, and takes the
form of excessive facial and body hair,
commonly with a male pattern of
distribution.

Acne

This is typically on the face, but can also
affect the chest, shoulders and back.

Subfertility

If your periods are consistently irregular or
absent, the chances are ovulation is irregular
or not occurring at all. If this is the case, a
delay in conceiving is not uncommon. Being
diagnosed with PCOS does not mean you are
infertile. Many women with PCOS conceive
without any problems; some women find it
a little harder to get pregnant but manage
without medical intervention; others find
they need the help of fertility treatment,
whether drug-based or just by using
nutritional or natural therapies.

Weight problems

Women with PCOS can have problems losing
weight, as discussed in Chapters 1 and 7.

Hair loss   Male-pattern hair loss commonly occurs with thinning from the top or crown of the head, together with loss from the front and a receding hair line.

WHAT TREATMENTS ARE AVAILABLE?

Don't be afraid to ask why your doctor is prescribing a particular medication for you, or how it works. The most commonly prescribed medications are outlined below. Remember that you don't need to accept the first prescription or suggestion your doctor gives you. Ask if there are any other options. You may also decide to try and deal with the condition yourself, without drugs. Remember: whether you decide to take drugs or to use non-drug therapies, following the diet and exercise advice in this book will be of enormous value.

Treatment for Irregular Periods

The mainstay of treatment for irregular periods has been the combined oral contraceptive pill, which is not helpful if you are trying for a baby. The treatment takes over the control of your menstrual cycle by overriding the production of your hormones. It also decreases the ovaries' production of testosterone and may result in a reduction of androgen-dependent symptoms such as acne and hirsutism, as well as regulating your cycle.

The problem with the Pill is that its long-term use can exacerbate insulin resistance, which may make your symptoms worse, particularly if you want to come off the Pill at a later date.

The British Medical Association's *Official Guide to Medicines and Drugs* says that synthetic oestrogens can trigger diabetes in susceptible individuals, which suggests it can increase insulin resistance and, as a result, weight gain. The Guide says, 'Oestrogens may also trigger the onset of diabetes mellitus in susceptible people, or aggravate blood-sugar control in diabetic women.'[5]

This exacerbation may make the Pill unsuitable for women who are already overweight.

Treatment of Excess Hair and Acne

Excess hair (hirsutism) and acne are treated using drugs which have been shown to have an anti-androgen action. The two most commonly prescribed are *cyproterone acetate* and *spironolactone*. They work by stopping the binding of the activated testosterone molecule to receptors on the skin and hair follicles. The effects take two or three months to appear, and are lost soon after stopping the treatment. Both drugs may actually make irregular periods worse and are contraindicated while trying to conceive. Cyproterone acetate is available in the combined oral contraceptive form called Dianette.

Treatment of Infertility

For those wishing to conceive, there are essentially three strategies:

1 To stimulate the ovaries to ovulate again, clomiphene citrate is often the first line of treatment. The drug carries with it a risk of multiple births (twins or triplets), and recent recommendations suggest that clomiphene should not be given for more than six cycles, as prolonged use can increase the risk of developing ovarian cancer in later life.
2 For those in whom colomiphene does not work, daily injections of follicle-stimulating hormone (FSH) are usually the next option. This injection program has a high success rate.
3 As an alternative to FSH treatment, or if this is not successful, some patients will move on to assisted connection techniques such as in-vitro fertilization (IVF).

Other PCOS symptoms tend to be ignored while these treatments are being tried, since the treatments mentioned either stop conception occurring or are not safe to be taken while pregnant.

Lowering Insulin Resistance

Metformin, a treatment often used to treat non-insulin-dependent diabetes, has been found to have uses in treating all of the classic symptoms of PCOS. It reduces insulin, testosterone and Luteinizing Hormone levels. These biochemical changes have been associated with a return to a regular menstrual cycle, ovulation, weight loss and a reduction in the symptoms of androgen excess.

It is important to remember, though, that all medications which offer benefits also have side-effects and contraindications. The list of current contraindications for Metformin includes endocrine disorders, infections, pregnancy, lactation and stress. However, dietary changes and lifestyle management are simple, safe, have no side-effects or contraindications and should be the first line of attack before you resort to drug treatments.

Complementary Therapies

Complementary therapies such as acupuncture, aromatherapy, homoeopathy, medical herbalism, nutritional therapy and reflexology are just some of the therapies which women with PCOS seem to find most helpful in dealing with their symptoms. The evidence in support of these treatments is anecdotal and comes from talking to women with PCOS and how they are managing their symptoms.

CAN PCOS BE CURED?

The symptoms of PCOS are all commonly associated with times of hormonal imbalance such as puberty, pregnancy and menopause. This has led to PCOS being generally classified as a gynaecological disorder.

Taking the contraceptive pill can help to even out irregular periods and mask some of the symptoms of PCOS. However, research done into PCOS has shown that women with the syndrome are at an increased risk of recurrent miscarriage and developing diabetes and heart disease. It seems that the hormonal symptoms are actually triggered off by a deeper underlying cause, which has long-term health consequences. The cysts and other symptoms of PCOS develop as a result of a genetic disposition towards PCOS, as well as environmental factors such as diet, lifestyle and stress levels.

One team of researchers has proposed that there's a male counterpart to polycystic ovaries in women: premature male-pattern baldness, defined as 'significant hair loss before the age of 30'.[6] And, according to recent research from St George's Hospital Medical School in London, male siblings of women with PCOS have an increased risk of insulin resistance and heart disease.

The general consensus is that there is no cure as such for PCO/S, because some women are born with a genetic predisposition or susceptibility for the condition. However, keeping the symptoms under control is within every woman's grasp. You can deal with the condition and help yourself to feel better by getting to grips with dietary and lifestyle changes to encourage hormonal balance. There are also specific treatments which target certain symptoms such as acne or excess hair.

There may be no cure for polycystic ovaries, but the condition does not have to destroy the quality of your life. If the cysts are a symptom of hormonal imbalance, as experts believe, balancing your hormones through the food you eat can help. Inevitably there will be times when you get down because you are stressed and are not eating well, and some symptoms such as spots and fatigue can resurface, but if you understand the basics of a healthy diet and how eating the wrong kinds of foods can make your PCOS symptoms worse, you can soon get back on track.

Many women find that with the right diet and exercise programme, symptoms disappear. If you find the prospect of a lifetime on a new eating regime daunting, remind yourself that if this means improved health and well-being, and a better quality of life, it is well worth the effort.

Suggested Reading

ACNE

Good Skin Doctor, Anne Lovell, Tony Chu (Thorsons)

Natural Beauty: Natural Approaches to Skin and Hair Care, Sidra Shaukat (Health Essentials)

ADDITIVES

E Is for Additives, Maurice Hanssen, Jill Marsden (Thorsons)

ALOPECIA (HAIR LOSS)

The Hair Loss Cure, Elizabeth Steele (Thorsons)

The Truth about Women's Hair Loss, Spencer Kobren (McGraw Hill)

ALTERNATIVE THERAPY

Alternative Medicine for Dummies, James Dillard and Terra Ziporyn (Dummies Press/IDG Books)

Alternative Therapy – The Definitive Guide, Burton Goldberg (Future Medicine Publishing Inc.)

The Hamlyn Encyclopedia of Complementary Therapies (Hamlyn)

Nine Ways to Body Wisdom, Jennifer Harper (Thorsons)

Women's Encyclopedia of Natural Medicine, Tori Hudson (McGraw Hill)

BODY IMAGE

Body Image Workshop, Thomas Cash (New Harbinger)

Self-esteem, Gael Lindenfield (Thorsons)

Self-esteem Companion, Matthew McKay (New Harbinger)

611 Ways to Boost Your Self-esteem, Bryan Robinson (Health Communications)

10 Days to Great Self-esteem, David Burns (Vermillion)

Transforming Body Image, Marcia Hutchinson (Crossing)

200 Ways to Love the Body You Have, Marcia Hutchinson (Crossing)

COOKBOOKS/RECIPES

Cooking Without, Barbara Cousins (Thorsons)

Food Combining for Health Cookbook, Jean Joice, Jackie Le Tissier (Thorsons)

The Good Carb Cookbook: Secrets of Eating Low on the GI, Sandra Woodruff (Avery)

Gourmet Prescription, Deborah Friedson Chud (Bay Books)

The Insulin Resistance Diet, Cheryl Hart (McGraw Hill)

The Low Carb Cookbook, Fran McCullough (Hyperion)

Low Carb Recipes Fast & Easy, Belinda Schweinhart (ASIN)

The Optimum Nutrition Cookbook, Patrick Holford (Piatkus)

The Sunday Times Vitality Cookbook, Susan Clarke (Harper Collins)

Vegetarian Cooking for People with Diabetes, Patricia Le Share (Book Publishing Co)

Vegetarian Cooking Without, Barbara Cousins (Thorsons)

Sophie Elkan

If you'd like to learn more about Sophie's recipes you can e-mail her at:

sophieelkan@yahoo.co.uk

DEPRESSION

Burned Out and Blue, Kristina Dowling Orr (Thorsons)

Climbing Out of Depression, Sue Atkinson (Lion Publishing)

Depression – with information on conventional and alternative approaches (Element's Natural Way series)

Overcoming Depression: What Therapy Doesn't Teach You and Can't Give You, Richard O'Connor (Berkley Publishing Group)

St John's Wort: Your Natural Prozac, Norman Rosenthal (Thorsons)

DETOX

Cleanse Your System, Amanda Ursell (Thorsons)

The Detox Manual, Suzannah Oliver (Pocket Books)

The Liver Cleansing Diet, Sandra Cabot (Women's Health Advisory Service)

The Living Beauty Detox Program, Ann Louise Gittleman (Harper San Francisco)

DIABETES/INSULIN RESISTANCE

Blood Sugar Blues: Overcoming the Hidden Dangers of Insulin Resistance, Miryam Ehrlich Williamson (Thorsons)

Coping with Diabetes, Robert Phillips (Avery)

Diabetes – with information on conventional and alternative approaches (Element's Natural Way series)

The Diabetes Cure, Vern S Cherewatenko (Thorsons)

Healthy Living with Diabetes, Margot Fromer (New Harbinger)

Syndrome X: Managing Insulin Resistance, Deborah Romaine (Harper)

Victory over Diabetes, William Philpott (Keats)

DIET/NUTRITION

The Carbohydrate Addict's Diet, Heller and Heller (New American Library)

The Food Combining Diet, Kathryn Marsden (Thorsons)

Food: Your Miracle Medicine, Jean Carper (Simon and Schuster)

The GI Factor, Anthony Leeds (Coronet)

Glucose Revolution: Guide to the Glycemic Index, Thomas Wolever (Marlowe)

Healing with Whole Foods, Paul Pitchford (North Atlantic)

Prescription for Nutritional Healing, James and Phyllis Balch (Avery)

Sugar Busters, H Leigton Stewart (Ballantine)

Syndrome X: Complete Nutritional Program for Insulin Resistance, Jack Challem (John Wiley)

EATING DISORDERS

The Eating Disorder Sourcebook, Carolyn Costin (McGraw Hill)

Eating Disorders – A Parent's Guide (Great Ormond Street Hospital Eating Disorders Clinic), Bryan Lask and Rachel Bryant-Waugh (Penguin)

Food for Thought: Sourcebook for Obesity and Eating Disorders, Diana Cassell (Facts on File)

Good Girls Do Swallow, Rachael Oakes-Ash (Mainstream Publishing)

The Hunger Within: A Twelve-week Self-guided Journey from Compulsive Eating to Recovery, Marilyn Migliore and Philip Ross (Doubleday)

When Women Stop Hating Their Bodies: Freeing Yourself from Food and Weight Obsession, Jane R Hirschmann and Carol H Munter (Ballantine/Fawcett)

FATIGUE

The Beat Fatigue Handbook, Erica White (Thorsons)

FERTILITY

The Fertility Sourcebook, M Sara Rosenthal (Lowell House)

Making a Baby: Everything You Need to Know to Get Pregnant, Debra Fulghum Brus and Samuel S Thatcher MD, PhD (Ballantine)

Planning for a Healthy Baby, Foresight (Vermillion)

In Pursuit of Fertility: A Fertility Expert Tells You How to Get Pregnant, Robert Franklin, Dorothy Brockman (Owl Books)

Taking Charge of Your Fertility, Toni Weschler (HarperPerennial)

What to Expect When You're Expecting, Arlene Eisenberg (Workman Publishing)

FITNESS BOOKS/VIDEOS

Be Your Best, Sally Gunnell (Thorsons)

Complete Book of Yoga, Vimla Lalvani (Hamlyn)

The Complete Illustrated Guide to Yoga, Howard Kent (Element)

Rosemary Conley fitness videos, BBC Worldwide and Video Collection Inc, VHS

Diets Don't Work, Vimla Lalvani, Lace International VHS

The Idiot's Guide to Fitness, Claire Walker (Alpha)

Introduction to Tai Chi, Lucy Lloyd-Barker, Inc Vision Ltd, VHS

Principles of Tai Chi, Paul Brecher (Thorsons)

FOOD AND MOOD

Feeding the Body, Nourishing the Soul, Deborah Keston (Conari)

Food and Mood, Elizabeth Somer (Owl Books)

The Food and Mood Handbook, Amanda Geary (Thorsons)

Women's Moods: What Every Woman Should Know About Hormones, the Brain and Emotional Health, Deborah Sichel (William Morrow)

Your Miracle Brain, Jean Carper (Thorsons)

GIVE-UP-SMOKING BOOKS

Breathe Easy: The Friendly Stop Smoking Guide For Women, Susannah Hayward (Penguin)

Allen Carr's Easy Way to Stop Smoking (Penguin)

Stop Smoking Naturally, Martha Work (Keats)

HERBAL MEDICINE

The Complete Woman's Herbal, Anne McIntyre (Henry Holt)

Herbal Defence, Robyn Landis (Thorsons)

The Herbal Menopause Book, Amanda Crawford (Crossing)

Herbal Remedies for Women, Amanda Crawford (Prima)

Vitex – the Woman's Herb, Christopher Hobbs (Botanica)

Woman Medicine – Vitex Agnus Castus, Simon Mills (Amberwood Publishing)

HORMONES

Androgen Disorders in Women: The Most Neglected Hormone Problem, Theresa Francis-Cheung, James Douglas (Hunter House)

Balancing Hormones Naturally, Kate Neil, Patrick Holford (Piatkus)

Before the Change: Taking Charge of Your Perimenopause, Anne Louise Gittleman (Harper SanFrancisco)

The Good News about Women's Hormones, Geoffrey Redmond (Warner)

Dr Susan Love's Hormone Book, Susan Love (Random House)

INFERTILITY

The Infertility Book, Carla Harkness (Celestial)

The Infertility Companion, Anna Furse (Thorsons)

Infertility: The Last Secret, Anna McGrail (Bloomsbury)

Infertility: a sympathetic approach to understanding the causes and options for treatment, Robert Winston (Vermillion)

Natural Solutions to Infertility, Marilyn Glenville (Piatkus)

NATURAL/WELL WOMAN

Body Foods for Women, Jane Clarke (Orion)

Complete Women's Health (Royal College of Obstetricians and Gynecologists)

8 Weeks to Optimum Health, Andrew Weil (Little Brown)

The Natural Health Handbook for Women, Marilyn Glenville (Piatkus)

Our Bodies Our Selves for the New Century, Boston Women's Health Collective (Touchstone)

Women's Bodies, Women's Wisdom, Christine Northrup (Bantam)

Women's Encyclopedia of Natural Medicine, Tori Hudson (McGraw Hill)

ORGANIC LIVING

Organic Living, Michael Van Staten (Frances Lincoln)

Organic Living: Simple Solutions for a Better Life, Lynda Brown (DK Publishing)

Organic Living in 10 Simple Lessons, Karen Sullivan (Barnes Ed)

Taste Life: The Organic Choice, David Richard (Vital Health)

PCOS

PCOS: A Woman's Guide to Dealing with Polycystic Ovary Syndrome, Colette Harris, Adam Carey (Thorsons)

PCOS, Gabor Kovacs (Cambridge University Press)

PCOS: The Hidden Epidemic, Samuel S Thatcher MD, PhD (Perspective Press)

STRESS

The Little Book of Calm, Paul Wilson (Penguin)

101 Shortcuts to Relaxation, Cathy Hopkins (Bloomsbury)

Stress, Anxiety and Insomnia, Michael Murray (Prima)

Stressbusters, Robert Holden (Thorsons)

Timeshifting, Stephen Rechstaffen (Vermillion)

Write Your Own Prescription for Stress, Kenneth Matheny (New Harbinger)

SUPPLEMENTS

Earl Mindell's Supplement Bible (Thorsons)

The Nutritional Health Bible, Linda Lazarides (Thorsons)

The Optimum Nutrition Bible, Patrick Holford (Piatkus)

Thorsons Complete Guide to Vitamins and Minerals, Leonard Mervyn (Thorsons)

THYROID

Thyroid Problems, Patsy Westcott (Thorsons)

Thyroid – Why Am I So Tired?, Martin Budd (Thorsons)

WEIGHT LOSS

Lighten Up, Pete Cohen, Judith Verity (Century)

The Zone: A Dietary Road Map to Lose Weight Permanently, Barry Sears (Harper Collins)

References

CHAPTER I

1 Sozen, I et al., 'Hyperinsulinism and its interaction with hyperandrogenism in polycystic ovary syndrome', *Ob and Gyn Survey* 55 (5) (May, 2000): 321–8; Dunaif, A, 'Insulin action in the polycystic ovary syndrome', *Endocrinology and Metabolism Clinics of North America* 28 (2) (June, 1999): 341–59

2 Kiddy, D S et al., 'Differences in clinical and endocrine features between obese and non-obese subjects with polycystic ovary syndrome: an analysis of 263 cases', *Clin Endocrin* 32 (1989): 213–20

3 Clark A et al., 'Weight loss results in significant improvement in pregnancy and ovulation rates in anovulatory obese women', *Human Reproduction* 10 (1995): 2705–12

4 Kiddy, D S et al., 'Improvement in endocrine and ovarian function during dietary treatment of obese women with polycystic ovary syndrome', *Clin Endocrin* 36 (1992): 105–11

5 Hartz, A et al., 'The association of obesity with infertility and related menstrual abnormalities in women', *International Journal of Obesity* 3 (1979): 57–73

6 Evans, D J et al., 'Relationship of androgenic activity to body fat topography, fat cell morphology and metabolic aberrations in premenopausal women', J Clin Endocrinol Metab 57 (1983): 304–10

7 Kovacs, Gabor T, Polycystic Ovary Syndrome (Cambridge University Press, 2000)

8 Robinson, S et al., 'Postprandial thermogenesis is reduced in polycystic ovary syndrome and is associated with increased insulin resistance', Clin Endocrin 36 (1992): 537–43

9 Legro, Richard, 'Polycystic Ovary Syndrome: Current and future treatment paradigms', Am J Obstet Gynecol 179 (1998): s94–100

10 Carmina, E and Lobo, R A, 'Polycystic ovary syndrome (PCOS) arguably the most common endocrinology is associated with significant morbidity in women', J Clin Endocrinol Metab 84 (6) (June 1999): 1897–9; Lobo, R A and Carmina, E, 'The importance of diagnosing the polycystic ovary syndrome', Annals of Internal Medicine 132 (12) (June 20, 2000): 989–93

11 Michelmore, K F, 'Polycystic ovaries and eating disorders – are they related?', Human Reproduction 16 (4) (2001): 765–9

12 Conway, G S, Agrawal, R, Betteridge, D J et al., 'Risk factors for coronary heart diseases in lean and obese women with polycystic ovary syndrome', Clin Endocrinology 37 (1992): 119–25

13 Rajkhowa, M, Glass, M R, Rutherland, A J, Michelmore, K and Balen, A H, 'Polycystic ovary syndrome: a risk for cardiovascular disease?', BJOG: An International Journal of Obstetrics and Gynecology 107 (1) (Jan, 2000): 11–18

14 Dahlgreen, E, Johansson, S, Lindstedt, G et al., 'Women with polycystic ovary syndrome wedge resection in 1956 to 1965: a long-term follow-up on natural history and circulation hormones', Fertility and Sterility 57 (1992): 505–13

15 Rajkhowa, M, Glass, M R, Rutherland, A J, Michelmore, K and Balen, A H, 'Polycystic ovary syndrome: a risk for cardiovascular disease?', BJOG: An International Journal of Obstetrics and Gynecology 107 (1) (Jan, 2000): 11–18

16 Schildkraut, J M, 'Epithelial ovarian cancer risk among women with PCOS', Obstetrics and Gynecology 88: 554–9

17 Spector, N et al., 'Cancer, genes and the environment', New England Journal of Medicine 343 (Nov 16, 2000): 1494–6

18 Polson, D W, Adams, J, Wadsworth, J and Franks, S, 'Polycystic Ovaries – a common finding in normal women', Lancet i (1988): 870–2; Franks, S, 'Polycystic ovary syndrome', New Engl J Med 333 (1995): 853–61

19 Taylor, Ann et al., 'Impact of diet composition on weight loss and endocrine parameters in women with PCOS', Rep Endocrine Unit, Mallinkkrodt General Clinical Research Center, Massachusetts General Hospital, Boston, MA, Androgen Disorders in Women Poster session (2000) 6/21, Board 433

CHAPTER 2

1 Jenkins D J A et al., 'Glycemic Index of foods', J Clin Nutr 46 (supplement 2; 132; 1978): 386–93

2 Wild, R A, Painter, P C, Coulson, P B et al., 'Lipoprotein lipid concentrations and cardiovascular risk in women with polycystic ovary syndrome', J Clin Endocrinol Metab 61 (1985): 946–51; Conway, G S, Agrawal, R, Betteridge D J et al., 'Risk factors for coronary artery disease in lean and obese women with polycystic ovary syndrome', Clin Endocrin 37 (1992): 119–25

3 Rajkhowa, M, Glass, M R, Rutherford, A J, Michelmore, K and Balen, A H, 'Polycystic Ovary Syndrome: A risk factor for cardiovascular disease?', Br J Obstet Gynaecol 10 (2000): 11–18

4 Dahlgreen, E, Johansson, S, Lindstedt, G et al., 'Women with Polycystic Ovary Syndrome wedge resection in 1956 to 1965: A long-term follow up on natural history and circulation hormones', *Fertility and Sterility* (1992): 505–13

CHAPTER 3

1 Hikon, H et al., 'Antihepatotoxic actions of flavonolignans from Silybum marianum fruits', *Planta Medica* 50 (1984): 248–50

2 Stanton, C and Gray, R, 'Effects of caffeine consumption on delayed conception', *American Jour of Epidemiology* 142 (12) 1995: 1322–29

3 Hughes, J M et al., 'Hypothalamic-pituitary function in thirty-one women with chronic alcoholism', *Clinical Endocrinol* (Oxford) 12 (1980): 543–51; Valmake, M et al., 'Sex hormones in amenorrheaic women with alcoholic liver disease', *Journal of Clinical Endocrinology and Metabolism* 59 (1984): 133–8

4 Jensen, T et al., 'Does moderate alcohol consumption affect fertility? Follow-up study among couples planning pregnancy', *BMJ* 317 (1998): 505–10; Hakim, R et al., 'Alcohol and caffeine consumption and decreased fertility', *Fertility and Sterility* 70 (4) 1998: 632–7

5 Ingram, D J, *Journal of the National Cancer Institute* 79 (1987): 1225

6 Friends of the Earth press briefing for Safer Chemicals Campaign 'Chemicals and Health', www.foe.co.uk/resource/briefings/chemicals_and_health.pdf

7 Theuer, R, 'Effect of oral contraceptive agents on vitamin and mineral needs: a review', *J of Reproductive Med* 8 (1) (Jan 1972): 1320; Tyrer, L B, 'Nutrition and the pill', *J of Reproductive Med* 29 (7 suppl) (Jul 1984): 547–50

8 British Medical Association, *Official Guide to Medicines and Drugs* (Dorling Kindersley, 1998): 147

9 *Lancet* 354 (October 23, 1999): 1435–9

10 Dr Kurt Kraichin *et al.* at the Sleep Laboratory of the University of Basel, Switzerland, as published in *Nature* 401 (September 2, 1999): 36–7

CHAPTER 5

1 Kelly *et al.*, 'Psychodynamic Psychological Correlates with Secondary Amenorrhea', *Psychosomatic Medicine* 16 (1954): 129; Piotrowski, T, 'Psychogenic Factors in Anovulatory Women', *Fertility and Sterility* 13 (1962): 11

2 D E Stewart *et al.*, 'Infertility and eating disorders', *American Journal of Obstetrics and Gynecology* 163 (1990): 1196–9; Dawson, D W, 'Infertility and Folate Deficiency', *British Journal of Obstetrics and Gynecology* 89 (1982): 678

3 Vigersky, B A *et al.*, 'Hypothalamic dysfunction in secondary amenorrhea associated with simple weight loss', *New England Journal of Medicine* 297 (1977): 1141–5

4 Kovacs, Gabor T (ed), *Polycystic Ovary Syndrome* (Cambridge University Press, 2000)

5 Kiddy, D S *et al.*, 'Differences in Clinical and Endocrine features between obese and non-obese subjects with PCOS: an analysis of 263 cases', *Clinical Endocrinol* 32 (1990): 213–20

6 Study published in *Archives of Dermatology*, December 1998

CHAPTER 6

1 Willett, Walter, MD, Professor of Epidemiology and Nutrition at the Harvard School of Public Health, Harvard Medical School, in *Journal of the American Medical Association* February 12, 1997

2 Salmerón, Jorge *et al.*, 'Dietary fat intake and risk of Type II diabetes in women', *American Journal of Clinical Nutrition* June 2001

3 *Stroke* (a journal of the American Heart Association), March 3, 2000 and June 7, 2000

4 Madar, Abel, Sarnish and Arad, 'Glucose-lowering effect of fenugreek in non-insulin-dependent diabetics', *European Journal of Clinical Nutrition* 42 (1998): 51–4; Al-Habari and Rahan, 'Antidiabetic and hypocholesterolemic effects of fenugreek', *Phytotherapy Research* 12 (1998): 233–42

CHAPTER 7

1 Kiddy, D S *et al.*, 'Differences in Clinical and Endocrine features between obese and non-obese subjects with PCOS: an analysis of 263 cases', *Clin Endocrin* 32 (1990): 213–20

2 Robinson, Stephen *et al.*, 'Postprandial thermogenesis is reduced in polycystic ovary syndrome and is associated with increased insulin resistance', *Clin Endocrin* 36 (1992): 537–43

3 Collins *et al.*, announced at the 13th International Congress of Dietetics, Edinburgh, Scotland, 2000

4 Eckel, Dr Robert H, senior author of advisory paper for the American Heart Association, March 20, 2001

5 Eckel, Dr Robert H et al. (American Heart Association's Nutrition Committee), 'High protein diets not proven', *Circulation* October, 2001

6 Anderson, Dr Torben and Fogh, J, Charlottenlund Medical Centre, Denmark

7 British Medical Association, *Official Guide to Medicines and Drugs* (Dorling Kindersley, 1998): 147

8 University of Southern California School of Medicine research study 'Mini-pill increases risk of Diabetes', *Journal of the American Medical Association* Aug 12, 1998

9 'Nutrition and the pill', *Journal of Rep Med* 29 (7) (July 1984): Suppl 547–50

10 Theuer, Richard, 'Effect of oral contraceptives agents on vitamin and mineral needs: a review' *Journal of Rep Med* 8 (1) (Jan 1972)

CHAPTER 8

1 Propping, D and Katzorke, T, 'Treatment of corpeus luteum insufficiency', *Zeitschr Allgemeinmedizin* 63 (1987): 932–3

2 Dittmar, F et al., 'Premenstrual Syndrome: Treatment with a phytopharmaceutical', *T W Gynakol* 5 (1) 1992: 60–8

3 Bunyapraphatsara, N et al., 'Antidiabetic activity of aloe vera L juice: Clinical trial in diabetes mellitus patients', *Phytomedicine* 3 (3) (1996): 245–8

4 American Diabetes Association 32nd Research Symposium: 'The Role of Oxidants and Antioxidant Therapy in Diabetic Complications', Orlando, Florida, Nov. 15–17, 1996

5 Lefebvre, P et al., 'Influences of weight, body fat patterning and nutrition on the management of PCOS', *Human Reproduction* 12 Suppl 1 (Oct 1997): 72–81

6 Kidd, G S et al., 'The effects of pyridoxine on pituitary hormone secretion in amenorrhea-galactorrhea syndrome', *Journal of Clin Endocrinol and Metabolism*, 54 (4) (1982): 872–5

7 Pramik, J-J, 'Study says chromium supplement helps some diabetics', *Medical Tribune News Service*, June 11, 1996

8 Evans, G W et al., 'Composition and biological activity of chromium-pyridine carbosylate complexes', *Journal of Inorganic Biochemistry* 49 (1993): 177–87

9 Van Gall, L et al., 'Biochemical and clinical aspects of co-enzyme Q10', *Journal of Vitaminology* 4 (1984): 369; Shiega, Y et al., 'Effect of co-enzyme Q10 treatment on blood sugar and ketone bodies of diabetics', *Journal of Vitaminology* 12 (1966): 293–8

10 Behme, M T, 'Dietary fish oil enhances insulin sensitivity in miniature pigs', *Journal of Nutrition* 126 (1996): 1549–53; Storlien, L H, et al., 'Dietary fats and insulin action', *Diabetologia* 39 (1996): 621–31

11 Tarin, J et al., 'Effects of Maternal aging and dietary anti-oxidants supplements on ovulation, fertilization and embryo development in vitro in the mouse', *Reproduction Nutrition, Development* 38 (5) (1998): 499–508

12 Madar, Abel, Sarnish and Arad, 'Glucose-lowering effect of fenugreek in non-insulin-dependent diabetics', *European Journal of Clinical Nutrition* 42 (1998): 51–4; Al-Habari and Rahan, 'Antidiabetic and hypocholesterolemic effects of fenugreek', *Phytotherapy Research* 12 (1998): 233–42

13 Rushton, D H et al., 'Letter to Ferritin and fertility', Lancet 337 (1991): 1554

14 Szekely, Dr E B, 'The essene way', Journal of Biogenic Living (US International Biogenic Society, 1978)

15 American Diabetics Association, 'Magnesium supplementation in the treatment of diabetes', Diabetes Care 15 (1992): 1065–7

16 Wagner, H, in J L Beal and E E Reinhards (eds), Natural Products as Medicinal Agents (1981)

17 Linde, Klaus et al., British Medical Journal 313 (1996): 253–8

18 Journal of Nutrition 125 (1995): 437–45

19 Messina, M, 'Increasing use of soyfoods and their potential role in cancer prevention', Perspectives in Practice 7 (1991): 836–40; Dwyer, J et al., 'Tofu and soy drinks contain phytoestrogens', J Am Det Assoc 94 (7) (1994): 739–43; Beckman, N, 'Phytoestrogens and compound that affect estrogen metabolism – part 2', Aust J Med Herbalism 7 (2) (1995): 27–33

20 Cassidy, A et al., 'Biological effects of a diet of soy protein rich in isoflavones on the menstrual cycle of premenopausal women', American Journal of Clinical Nutrition 60 (1994): 333–40

21 Harland, B F and Harden-Williams, B A, 'Is vanadium of human nutritional importance yet?', Journal of the American Dietetic Association 94 (1994): 891–4

CHAPTER II

1 Wurtzman, Judith J, Managing Your Mind and Mood Through Food (New York: Rawson Associates, 1986): 7

2 Piotrowski, T, 'Psychogenic Factors in Anovulatory Women', *Fertility and Sterility* 13 (1962): 11; Loftus, T, 'Psychogenic factors in anovulatory women: behavioral and psychoanalytic aspects of anovulatory amenorrhea', *Fertility and Sterility* 13 (1962): 20; E Stewart *et al.*, 'Infertility and Eating Disorders', *American Journal of Obstetrics and Gynecology* 163 (1990): 1196-9

3 Jahanfar, E, Eden *et al.*, 'Bulimia nervosa and polycystic ovary syndrome', *Gynecol Endocrinol* 9 (1995): 113-17

4 Michelmore, K F, 'Polycystic ovaries and eating disorders: are they related?', *Human Reproduction* 16 (4) (2001): 765-9

APPENDIX

1 Adams, J, Polson, D W and Franks, S, 'Prevalence of polycystic ovaries in women with anovulation and idiopathic hirsutism', *BMJ* 293 (1986): 355-9

2 Stein, I F and Leventhal, M L, 'Amenorrhea associated with bilateral polycystic ovaries', *Am J Obstet Gynecol* 29 (1935): 181-91

3 Franks, S, Gharani, N, Watermouth, D M, Batty, S, White, D, Williamson, R and McCarthy, M, 'The genetic basis of polycystic ovary syndrome', *Human Reproduction* 12 (1997): 2641-8

4 Polson, D W, Adams, J, Wadsworth, J and Franks, S, 'Polycystic Ovaries – a common finding in normal women', *Lancet* i (1988): 870-2

5 British Medical Association, *Official Guide to Medicines and Drugs* (Dorling Kindersley, 1998): 147

6 Carey, A H, Chan, K L, Short, F, White, D M, Williamson, R and Franks, S, 'Evidence for a single-gene effect in polycystic ovaries and premature male pattern baldness', *Clin Endocrin* 38 (1993): 653-8

Index